A Whole New You

To Your Good Health

Laura Koenig Rivkin, B.S., CHHC, AADP, CPT

A Whole New You, To Your Good Health

To contact the publisher, visit www.awholenewyou.org

To contact the author, visit www.awholenewyou.org

ISBN 978-0-9962291-0-4

Library of Congress Control Number: 2015906601

Printed in the United States of America

Dedication

While writing this book, two important people in my life passed on.

I would like to dedicate this book in part to them:

Lynn Borders Caldwell, my college roommate, never stopped pursuing life to the fullest. She had courage, strength, and perseverance. I will never forget the good times we had.

Jack Kahn, my stepfather, had a wonderful sense of humor, amazing strength inside and out, determination, and the ability to always look at the positive in his life. He was an inspiration to me and to my family.

I also want to dedicate this book to some of my relatives who have passed on and are greatly missed.

To my cousin Marv. He was wise, a great cook (check out his recipe), and always made the holidays so special.

To my cousin and friend Debbie. She was beautiful inside and out, with a talent that stretched to the arts and beyond.

To my Aunt Bea. She was talented as an artist and a free spirit.

To my grandfather George. He was kind, caring, and a world ping pong champion! Your stories will never be forgotten!

To my grandmother Irene. She was one of the closest people to me. She taught me about life: how to love, take care of oneself, cook, and more!

To my father Samuel. Not a day goes by that I don't think of him. His kind, caring, and loving ways have passed on to me and my children. I am blessed to have had him as my father, even though it was for only a short while.

Table of Contents

Chapter 7

Chapter 8

Chapter 9

Chapter 10

Acknowledgements

A special thank you to the following individuals whose contributions and support made this book possible:

To my editor Tracey Kocz—Thank you for diligently working hard and under a tight deadline! Your kindness, thoughtfulness, and caring ways are greatly appreciated!

To my graphic designers, Roni Murillo—Thank you for all your hard work, dedication, and creativity. Your talents shine almost as much as you do! I am thrilled we connected in more ways than one. Thanks also to Carlene who, at the last minute, came through and put all the pieces of the book together. I am so grateful!

To Joshua, Lindsay, and the support from IIN—If it weren't for your encouragement, dedication, and support to keep us writing, I am not sure this book would exist! Thank you so much for all!

To John Calabrese—Your knowledge, support, guidance, patience, understanding, and encouragement have brought me to where I am today. I am forever grateful and blessed.

To K. Tukman—Your support, encouragement, wisdom, and insight are gifts I will always cherish. Thank you.

To my friends who supported me through it all:

Pauline, a sister at heart, confidante, and special person in my life. Thank you for supporting me always. I am so grateful to have you in my life!

Shari, your strength, guidance, loving and caring ways, as well as our long-term friendship have meant more to me than words can say.

Sylvia, my soul sister. Your inner strength, wisdom, and support are gifts I cherish. I am so thankful for our friendship!

Laura, thank you for being a wonderful friend and confidante. You have truly inspired me to write this book!

Alma, your encouragement, advice, and friendship have helped me through it all!

Lori, my friend and former college suitemate. Life reconnected us, and I am truly grateful! Thanks for all your input and support!

Kathy, your friendship, support, and all the books we read truly inspired me to write this one! Thank you for jumping in to take some last-minute pics, as well.

Julia, thank you for trusting and believing in me! Your kindness and caring ways make you special.

Jim, thank you for all your wisdom and guidance always. You are a true gem!

Mike, your support, guidance, and encouragement have meaning beyond words. I am blessed to know you.

Mitch, thank you for being a great influence and support system.

Tom, your knowledge and teachings have been a true gift. Namaste.

Roy, thank you for your patience, encouragement, understanding, and kindness. Thank you also for being the makeshift photographer! I am deeply grateful to have you in my life!

Thanks to My Family

My Uncle Eddy and Aunt Anna, Cousins Arlene, Bob and Jeanette, Jeff and Elissa, David, Karen and David, Brian and Katy, Amy and Carolina, Jeff and Felecia, David and Amy, Jane and Andy, Rich, Barbara and all their respective children:

Thank you all for your inspiration, support, and believing in me! I am grateful and blessed to have you in my life! Love you all!

A Special Note of Acknowledgement

To my mom Florette and sister Lisa—Thank you for your love, guidance, and support always. It is truly appreciated. Your encouragement to keep pushing forward has worked! Love you both!

To my two wonderful children, Eric and Elana—You are my most precious assets. There is no greater joy in my life than the both of you! I love you both with all my heart and more. May this book be an inspiration to you!

Although space precludes me from mentioning all the wonderful teachers, family members, friends, and clients who have touched my life in some way, you know who you are, with love and gratitude.

Prologue

I was inspired to write this book because I realize many people are so busy with their fast-paced lives—working, taking care of the kids, attending activities and meetings, and so on—that they forget to prioritize their own health! I was a busy single mom raising two very young children (ages 3 and 5) who had to do it all and work part-time to make ends meet. However, I still managed to squeeze in time for myself each day, even if only for 10 minutes. Taking time for yourself is so important no matter how busy you are. Granted, I struggled on occasion to make that time, but as the years went by, I realized if I did not set aside at least 10 minutes a day to focus on myself, what good was I to my children or to myself? It's easy to get caught up in the day-to-day routine and forget about yourself in the process. That's when you need to stop and say, "Wait a minute, I count here, too!" And that's exactly what I did. Yes, in some ways, it was more work. I cooked differently for myself than I did for my kids, as my dietary needs were different. I needed to eat properly to nourish my body, while gradually introducing my food choices to my children. I shopped at various health food stores. Fortunately, there has been a gradual progression of supermarkets offering healthier food options, which has made things a bit easier over time. No matter how little time I had, I made food shopping, prepping, and cooking a priority. My kids never really ate at fast food restaurants, and did not miss it anyway. They did have occasional junk food, but not on a daily basis.

Unfortunately, we all know too many people—family members, friends, coworkers—who are overweight, have diabetes or high blood pressure, or who have more serious illnesses, including cancer. Many people are dying younger these days, and I believe stress and not making the time to optimize their health are contributing to the cause. Hippocrates said, "Let Food Be Thy Medicine" and I believe this is so true. Food truly can heal the body if you allow the time for it to do so. Heart attacks are caused by poor eating—plain and simple. They are known as the "silent killer." Do you want to be part of that statistic or do you want to do something about your health once and for all?

Getting Out of Your Own Way

Countless people have said to me, "I know what I need to do. I just don't have time to do what is necessary to achieve optimal health."

Take a moment to reflect upon the above statement and then answer these questions:

1. Are you making excuses for yourself year after year and not really achieving your goal(s)?

   _____

   _____

2. What do you think holds you back?

   _____

   _____

3. Do you think it is more work than it's worth? If so, what is your self-worth?

   _____

   _____

4. What if you were given only six months to live? Would you find the time then to care about your own health?

   _____

   _____

If you answered yes to the last question, then live today as if it were getting close to that time frame, because we really never know when our time on this earth will be up. Preparing now, not when it's too late, is imperative! Kick yourself in the rear, get back on the horse, and let's get moving!

No More Excuses!

Introduction

My Story

I've been struggling with my health since the day I was born, literally. I was born a fighter and survivor. I truly feel my purpose in life is to pass on the knowledge I have gained in various facets of my life, especially related to health and well-being.

I was an Rh-negative baby and needed a blood transfusion at birth. I was also jaundiced. My father saw that I was turning blue, and by alerting the nurse and doctor, he saved my life. A few years later, I needed braces on my feet because I walked pigeon-toed. Years later, just after the start of puberty, I was diagnosed with scoliosis, which was not checked regularly at school at the time. I ended up wearing a Milwaukee brace for three years to help stabilize my curve. When it was time to remove the brace, my orthopedic doctor recommended I start weight training to help strengthen my back. Being young and adventurous, I found it fun and something to look forward to a few times a week. I never overexercised. I just worked on strengthening my muscles and helping to stop my curve from progressing further.

Over the years, I've had various ailments, such as severe acne (including boils on my skin), migraine headaches, allergies, digestive issues, and chronic fatigue. I was raised by a single mother after I lost my dad tragically at age 10. My mother did not understand health very well, other than going to the doctor and getting medication to fix the issue quickly. Little did she or I know that my body was extremely sensitive to each and every medication. My body developed many sensitivities and suffered many side-effects, one worse than the other. At one point in my late teens, I got frustrated with being sick and having more side-effects and ailments than I originally started with, so I decided to fight back. I decided to take control of my life and started fighting for it again in the best way I knew how.

I was always interested in health, as I used to go to a local health food store in my neighborhood starting at age 15. I taught myself how to read labels, what to look for, and was always curious. Since that time, I have been a health researcher on what the real truth is about optimal health and well-being. While doing some research, I became aware that my digestive issues were more severe than I had realized. As I got older, I noticed my abdomen often would be bloated, and, at times, it looked as though I was three months pregnant when I wasn't. After going to many doctors through the years,

I finally found one that could help me. She suggested I go on a gluten-free diet, which I did, even though it was difficult at first. I also started to change my diet a bit more and eliminated some foods to which my body didn't seem to react well. In those days, gluten-free and food allergies were not as common as they are today. Doctors thought my symptoms were all in my head. I felt alone and lost but kept forging ahead. I knew my symptoms were real, as I was not feeling well most of the time! Although I changed my diet, it still was not enough. I needed to go further in my research and get to the heart of my problem. Eventually, I found out that the issue stemmed from my childhood when I was put on many, many medications—one overlapping the other—used as a quick fix for one condition on top of another. Unfortunately, the medicines affected my gut health. As the years went on, I realized I was suffering from intestinal permeability, which is also known as leaky gut syndrome. This basically means that whatever I should have been digesting was actually leaking throughout my body and not digesting in my small intestine. I also developed something called small intestinal bacteria overgrowth, or SIBO. This means that I have more bad bacteria growing in my gut than good bacteria. Despite the fact that my diet is extremely healthy, bacteria like to feed on certain healthy foods, which unfortunately creates more bad bacteria. It has become a vicious cycle in my battle to get back to good health. (For those interested, I plan to write my next book on digestive health and my healing.)

There is a lot of misinformation and confusion out there. I hope to explain to you in simple terms how important it is to take control of your own health and make it a priority, no matter what. I've been through a lot in my lifetime and hope to save you the years of struggle I went through by giving you some of the information and knowledge I have learned over many years.

I was inspired to write this book based on information I was hearing from my clients, my family, and the public. I kept hearing over and over again that people want to get healthy but simply don't have the time! The alarm went off in my head, and I felt a longing to reach out to others. So here goes…

Chapter 1

Why Making Time for Your Health Is Important

Focusing on Ourselves Is Difficult

If you want to live a long, healthy life, some lifestyle changes may be necessary. The hardest thing for a parent, grandparent, caregiver, or even a health care practitioner to do is to focus on themselves. We were raised to take care of our family (or our patients in the case of a practitioner) first by either being the bread winner or the caregiver of the family and home. More women are entering the workforce today, and that means even less family time is available to them, which is especially true for working mothers.

The pace of our lifestyle in the U.S. is especially fast. We run around with our children after work, going from school to one or more activities, almost daily. Or we stay late at work because layoffs or cutbacks have forced us to work longer hours. Or we are a health care practitioner who gives of ourselves to others, working 10 or more hours daily.

Given the added stress in our lives, how do we find time to truly take care of **ourselves** each day?

Our Health Is Our Wealth

Not being able to find the time for ourselves each day is a bigger issue than we all might realize. "Our health is our wealth," and if we don't have it, we essentially have nothing. We want calmness, peace, and a stress-free environment in our lives. We want to be physically healthy and live a long, happy life. We want to see our children and grandchildren grow up. If we look at the model that Europeans follow, their lives are calmer and more peaceful, and they have less stress than Americans. Why is this? From a young age, Europeans are taught to take things slowly, eat their biggest meal at lunch, take naps during the day, and make time to relax and enjoy life. They make the time to take care of themselves consistently on a daily basis. This socially is their norm, whereas in the U.S., it is not.

What can we do as Americans to adopt some of the European philosophy? Statistics show that Europeans live longer, happier lives than we do. They eat healthier than we do, they laugh and enjoy life more than we do, and they are less stressed than we are.

As Americans, even though we have more freedom as a whole, do we really have freedom? We are taught to live under pressure, taught to live in a fast-paced environment, taught to eat the foods that are advertised the most, taught to follow the Standard American Diet (SAD), and taught to live in a materialistic society by keeping up with the Joneses. It's about living the American dream—living a life with freedom, wealth, a loving and happy family, a beautiful home with a white picket fence, and having all our dreams and wishes come true.

Important Questions to Think About

We are working harder and longer hours than ever, with less pay and/or benefits. Our expenses exceed our earnings. It seems most people cut down on food expenses more than any other expense. This is a mistake, because if we keep looking for the bargains and sale items, are we really nourishing our bodies optimally with the correct balance of nutrients on a daily basis?

Do we de-value our bodies on some level, feeling we are not worth the investment of optimal daily nourishment?

Are we valuing our materialistic possessions as more important than our own health and well-being? Are we forgetting about ourselves in body and mind? Do we tend to look at ourselves superficially, on the outside, wanting to look good for the world by portraying a certain style, image, or role?

Do we ever stop and think about taking care of the inside of our bodies at all? Is there even time to think in general about ourselves in relation to self-care and self-love?

It is important to stop and think, "If I had more time, more energy, and better health, wouldn't it be worth the effort?" Make your life worthwhile and meaningful. Put yourself first in ways that nourish your body and mind. To thrive and grow, this is essential.

Carving out time each day to take care of yourself in small increments is important. It can be just for 5–10 minutes at first. Here are some suggestions to get started:

Carving Out Time Each Day

Before starting your day

Take out a journal and write for a few minutes about what you are grateful for or what you are looking forward to this day.

Stretch your body, in or out of bed.

Drink a cup of warm herbal tea, sit and relax.

Take a deep breath, wake up slowly, and perhaps just sit and look out the window or at a calming picture.

Other Times of the Day

Between 4–6 pm

Take a break at work. Take a walk around the office or floor. Take some deep breaths. Stretch at your desk (see exercises at desk). Drink some water or herbal tea.

Try to avoid caffeine and unhealthy snacks at this time. This time of day is when our blood sugar tends to drop, energy gets low, and cravings begin.

Eat a healthy snack (see healthy snack list, pages 62–63).

Driving home from work

Listen to calming music, drink water, don't stress over traffic.

Dinnertime

Dinner does not have to be stressful. Planning ahead will help keep stress down. When coming home to your family from a hard day at work, have your spouse, partner, friend, or children help in prepping dinner. This way, you can give yourself 5–10 minutes to get settled. Then you can welcome all and get started with the evening.

By practicing some of these suggestions, you will feel a bit more relaxed and mindful of yourself. I recommend that you try these or add some of your own to start and end each day.

Bear in mind that taking care of yourself does not include fading out mindlessly by watching TV or surfing the internet. These are mindless distractions that actually stop us from performing the task(s) at hand. I am not saying that you should never watch TV or surf the internet. I am saying minimize the time you spend doing these activities. They can be for relaxation purposes, but they should not replace the inner work your body needs.

16 A Whole New You

Chapter 2

Taking Responsibility for Yourself and What That Means

It is imperative to truly focus on what is really going on inside ourselves. Most of us focus on others and/or the outside image of ourselves rather than the true essence of our being. Why? Perhaps it is easier and less emotionally charged. It is much easier to focus on others and to try to look good to someone else than it is for us to deal with what might really be going on for us deep inside.

Taking responsibility for yourself means going inside yourself. It means slowing down, having some quiet time, and checking in with what's going on for you at the time. Here are some ways to start taking responsibility for yourself:

1. *Journaling* is a wonderful way of getting in touch with yourself, because when you start to write, your true thoughts and feelings are down on paper and out of your mind and body. It is best to journal either at night before bedtime, or first thing when you wake up. Even writing down your dreams can help explore bottled-up emotions and stress that you might be holding onto without even realizing it. I highly recommend journaling to my clients, especially those who want to lose weight. It seems some people "hold on to the weight" they want to lose for safety and security. Journaling helps people release the hold and become free.

2. *Meditating, mindfulness practice, and yoga* also help you focus at the time. They help you get in touch with yourself and calm your mind and body. These helpful modalities will be discussed in more detail later in the book. I know of a wonderful free phone app called "Calm." It is quite useful for both beginners and advanced meditators. There is a guided meditation option that allows you to listen from 2 minutes up to 30 minutes while looking at beautiful scenery of your choice. There is another option that breaks this down into 7 steps, and you can listen to each step separately.

3. *Speak to a loved one or friend for support if you are having a difficult time.* Being responsible for yourself is probably even more difficult if you are a parent or a caregiver, as they tend to focus on "taking care" of everyone else before themselves. Time then seems to run out to take care of you! Don't make the

same mistake I did of putting my family first for years and forgetting about myself in the process! Yes, I exercised and went to the gym, ate healthy foods, and had some support from friends/family. However, deep down, I didn't take care of myself the way I should have. It's much more than just doing things quickly to get them done and then going on to the next thing on your list. I was always good at accomplishing many things at once. I was the master at multitasking! What? Slow down? It wasn't in my vocabulary. When you are used to going full speed ahead, living in a fast-paced environment, and keeping up with all you have to do and then some, how do you slow down? The first step is to be proactive toward your own health. Hit the brakes a bit, slow down, and ask yourself, "Does this really need to get done today?" Prioritize, and don't make a laundry list so long that nothing ends up getting accomplished. Start with a list of three of the most important items. Focus on only those three things, and if you end up with spare time during the day, then you can add one or two more items. Otherwise, you can just add those items to the next day's agenda and so on.

4. *If you're having health issues,* it might be worthwhile to take the information from your doctor and do your own research. Compare the information and formulate what might truly resonate for you in terms of healing your own body. Sometimes, we put too much faith into information that is given to us, and we don't advocate for ourselves and our own healing. Make yourself a priority when it comes to self-care. You need to count, no matter how busy you are.

5. *Energy Drainers.* It is important to distance yourself from negative people, also known as energy drainers. Energy drainers wear your body down and make you feel worse than you otherwise might feel. Take a look at the people in your life: Do they make you feel good? Do they support you when you need support? Or, do they look to you for support without listening to your needs? Do they take up so much of your time that you can't find downtime for yourself? If so, then perhaps you need to take a careful look at those relationships and examine why they are still in your life. As we grow as individuals, our own wants and needs change, and so, too, do the people we want in our lives. It might be difficult to let go of certain friends who have been in your life for a long time. However, if they don't serve you in a positive way, then they are not "healthy" for you. Consider parting ways and surround yourself instead with friends that support your growth and well-being. It would also be very difficult to let go of a partner/lover/companion. However, ask yourself, "Am I in this relationship to serve the other more than myself? Is he or she supportive, helpful, wanting to grow, fun to be with, and making me happy?" If not, then you might consider letting them go, as well, and seeking out a new partner or companion.

6. ***Eat clean, unprocessed whole foods.*** Our bodies generally don't thrive well on processed foods. They lack important nutrients that our body truly needs. Processed foods are modern day foods that are refined. Anything in a box or bag in the supermarket usually is processed, including bakery items made with flours and sugar. We tend to fill our body and mind with lots of tasty foods to satisfy our desires, emotions, and stresses. However, it's important to stop and think:

Am I satisfying my daily nutritional requirements?

How many vegetables/fruits per day do I have? (Make sure you limit fruit to no more than 2–3 servings per day. Having more than this amount is too much sugar for your body. It is best to eat more vegetables over fruit. However, opt for fruit over a sugary piece of candy.) Hint: include a minimum of 5 servings of vegetables per day.

How many meals do I have per day?

_____

How many processed snacks do I have per day? (Be honest.)

_____

If I eat whole foods, will that reduce my symptoms for high blood pressure, high cholesterol, diabetes, arthritis, cancer, and so on? This question is probably the most important to think about.

_____

What if my symptoms were reduced? How would that make me feel physically and emotionally?

_____

It might sound strange to think that whole foods can actually reduce symptoms and possibly heal the body of diseases, but various studies have shown this to be true. Whole foods contain fiber, vitamins, minerals, and antioxidants. When you eat whole foods, you are eating much more balanced, nutrient-dense foods that contain most (if not all) of the vitamins your body requires daily. Whole foods get absorbed into the body more easily than do supplements.

Make Your Life Worthwhile and Meaningful

If you dread going to work every day and are simply going through the motions for a paycheck, you might want to consider changing jobs or careers. Why spend so much time each day doing something that makes you unhappy? This unhappiness can carry over into your personal and family life. Of course, I'm not suggesting you leave your job until you have a plan of action. Perhaps just start to think about a few questions:

If I could do something else that would truly make me happy, fulfilled, and able to pay the bills, what would that be?

What can I contribute to others and society as a whole?

What is my passion(s)?

Just jot down ideas to start, even if you have a few moments at work when you are really feeling the dread. Think out of the box and let your thoughts and ideas flow. Even if you are middle aged or beyond, it's not too late. You can take many online courses today. Don't doubt your abilities even if your skills are limited. Making small, incremental changes ultimately can get you to where you want to go in life. It's the thought that starts the change. Getting out of your own way by not overthinking things and by doing more will help you get the ball rolling. You won't be able to progress to where you ultimately want to be if you get stuck in your old ways and comfort zone. As mentioned previously, if you are not happy with your friends or relationships, take a look at why and make some changes here, as well. It's really up to you to take control of your true happiness by pursuing a meaningful and worthwhile career, friendships, relationships, and family life.

Chapter 3

Emotional Blocks

An emotional block occurs when a person consciously or subconsciously decides not to deal with the emotions that arise from a negative experience. Some methods of blocking unpleasant experiences include suppression, shutting down, ignoring the experience, forgetting what happened, avoidance, and many others. These provide temporary relief, but the emotional blocks can build up inside us and become buried for years.

Examine whether you're stuck in old patterns. Do you tend to hold on to the past? If so, what do you think is holding you back? Is it a relationship that ended that you can't get past? Is it a friend or family member that didn't treat you the way you needed or desired to be treated? Is it hard for you to get in touch with your emotions? Sometimes, we swallow our pain without processing it at the time. The pain is then hidden from others, and we go through each day wearing a "false face." No one truly knows what we're thinking or feeling unless we're able to express and show our true self, not only to others, but most importantly, to ourselves. I realize this is easier said than done. Focusing on looking good for others through external appearance, financial status and so on stops you from showing your true self, so we end up putting on our mask daily. This, in turn, stops us from moving forward, and we get stuck and hide or avoid what we really need to focus on.

Sometimes, we're afraid to go forward, so we hold back without even realizing it. The word "fear" really is an acronym that means "False Evidence Appearing Real." Our thoughts, no matter how real they may seem to us at the time, might actually hold us back from pushing through our fear, which ultimately is what we want to do. I remember the book, *"Feel The Fear and Do It Anyway,"* by Susan Jeffers, Ph.D. It is so true. Picture in your mind's eye an image of yourself jumping through a hoop surrounded by fire, just like a lion would do at the circus. If you can get through to the other side of that hoop without too much thought, then you can conquer many of your fears. I felt stuck in my life for many years due to trauma in my childhood. I held on to the trauma, which held back my growth, daily thoughts, daily living, self-esteem, nourishment, etc. Consciously, I was not aware of this. I thought I was getting by just fine. Perhaps this was what I was willing to settle for back then. The turning point for me was probably when I had my first child. This made me see things a bit differently. If I am to care for another living being who is so fragile and in need of my love, support, daily care, encouragement, etc., then I better step up to the plate and push through my fear of being a new mother. That was the very beginning of my inner growth toward caring not only for my child, but also deeply for myself. Growth for me didn't stop there: it continued for the next 21 years. Writing this book and expressing part of myself to you, the reader, is the biggest hoop I have jumped through in letting go. I will continue to jump through hoops up until my last day on earth. Care to join me in growing?

When we think too much about what is holding us back, we actually hold ourselves back—the very thing we are trying not to do. Keeping things in your head, circling around and around, gets you nowhere. Try journaling when thoughts come to mind, or simply jot down the thought on a piece of paper wherever you are at the time. The idea is to get the thought down on paper and out of your mind so you can refer back to it at a later date. This will help you move forward from wherever you might be stuck in your life.

Often times, we get stuck in many areas of our life, not just one. If this is the case for you, focus on one area at a time. This way, you have a better chance of setting yourself up for success. Once you take care of that one area, you will be more motivated to take care of other areas in your life. For example, we might tell ourselves, "I need to lose weight." Why? Did someone tell you to? Is it a want or desire more than a need? When we need something, it comes from a place of "have to" almost out of desperation, fear, and stress. The very thing you want is not getting accomplished because of undue pressures from you or outside forces. Beating yourself up over it or procrastinating instead of following through are self-sabotaging ways of actually stopping yourself from reaching your goals.

Changing thought patterns can help with this. The more we overtalk, overthink, or overdo, the less likely we are to accomplish what we truly want to do. If you really want something, then go for it, and don't let anything get in your way. Get the support you need from friends and family, as well as from community support groups, whether in person or online. Many people tend to share their stories, and this can help resonate with what you might be going through. Practicing self-awareness, self-love, and self-acceptance of who you are and where you are at this moment is essential to lifting emotional blocks. I support you as you continue to learn, grow, and be the wonderful person you already are!

Chapter 4

Loving Yourself Inside and Out

What does it really mean to take care of yourself from the inside? It means don't focus on how you look or sound to others and don't worry about pleasing the outside world. Instead of being your true self, you might feel that you need to look good, sound good, and put on an act for others or even for yourself. Take a moment to reflect on this and ask yourself, "Am I always trying to impress my spouse, partner, friends, etc.? Do I put on a false face and image every day? Is wearing designer clothes and expensive jewelry, driving an expensive car, having a perfect home and being the right size and the right weight more important than my own self-image and being true to myself?" Think about why this might be and decide if you would like to explore the possibilities. Think of how you might treat a good friend. Then apply this to yourself. You matter in this world just as much as anyone, and you deserve to be who you are underneath all the cover-up. When we open up the door to the person we truly want to be (or already are but in hiding), it's almost as if a big cloud is being lifted, freeing us to be the person we were meant to be. The fear is gone, the blocks are lifted, and the growing process begins again.

Accept who you are today, not who or what you were in the past. Don't get down on yourself if you don't look the way you did 20 years ago. Most of us don't. That is reality. Accept the beautiful person you are and have always been. I know that it is easier said than done, but if you don't start taking the necessary steps toward healing and loving yourself on the inside, how will you grow and ultimately heal and care for yourself and your body? I used to pick on my imperfections rather than accept myself for who I was at the time. Like most people, I was focused more on the outside. I was a single mother of two kids under age 5 focused on their needs without allowing much time at all for myself. It took years to get to where I am today. I did somehow manage to make time to exercise (even if for only 20–30 minutes, 2–3 times per week), bringing my kids to the daycare at the gym. I also cooked healthy foods and, as my kids grew pickier, I sometimes ended up making three different meals almost daily! When I couldn't, I chose to buy the best foods on the go. You can do it now so you don't waste those precious years away!

Notice where you are in your life right now. Are you truly happy? Are you doing what you love to do? Do you have friends and family that are supportive? Are you anxious/stressed or relaxed and carefree? Take note, and if you feel anxious or stressed, what steps can you take today to become more relaxed? It's important to make slow, lasting lifestyle changes, rather than do things quickly or do nothing at all. Perhaps hiring a health coach could keep you on track. I teach my clients how to truly take care of themselves from the inside out with love and compassion. Here are some tips to follow:

1. Accept your body the way it is today. Don't change your body image for others. Look in the mirror and give yourself a hug each morning and night.

2. Throw away the scale. I know so many women who use the scale to judge their worth and image. Take charge of your eating patterns and lifestyle and try to incorporate daily exercise.

3. Journal each day or just jot down 3–5 positive things about you each day.

4. Find happiness in all you do. Even if it feels like a dark, dreary, depressing day, push through to find the silver lining of something happy and positive.

5. Smile more often. Look in the mirror and start your day with a smile. It helps even when you feel down.

6. Laugh. Laughter is the best medicine. It heals the body and takes away tension and stress. Watch a funny movie, go to a comedy show, or even watch a funny cartoon—whatever creates laughter for you.

7. Make daily functioning a priority. This includes eating healthier, getting more sleep, and relaxing your mind and body. By doing this, you will allow your body to get back into balance and you will feel much better overall!

8. Express your thoughts and emotions. Keeping them bottled up inside can cause more tension, physically and mentally, and can affect your overall health and well-being.

Weight Reduction Naturally

Avoid using the scale and counting calories. As stated above, the scale can hinder your self-worth and actually hold you back from weight loss. Calorie counting can do the same. Counting calories becomes an added stress over time and limits what you can/cannot eat and the amount. I believe that portion size of meals is important, as well. Wisely choose foods that will support your body type, genetic makeup, and lifestyle. Know the type of person you are when it comes to food. Are you an emotional eater? Do you eat when stressed? Are you so busy during the day that you skip meals and choose sugar or coffee to keep you going? Think of what you can choose to do instead of following typical old patterns. Eat more optimally by having a heart-healthy breakfast of clean protein, including vegetables, which might seem quite different, but they provide a good boost of energy to start your day. Substitute that candy bar or energy bar that's loaded with sugar with a piece of fruit instead that is naturally sweet.

Diets and calorie counting typically don't work for long periods of time. Have you ever experienced yo-yo dieting? When you diet, you either eliminate a food group or deprive yourself of something you really want. Over time, you will eat the very thing you were trying to avoid. Typically, people go on diets to lose weight fast due to an upcoming special event or to get ready for summer, or it's their New Year's resolution. Rushing to lose weight will only work temporarily, as you lose mostly water weight at the start. Diets only work for those who have a health condition that require a special diet, such as diabetes, digestive health issues, high blood pressure, etc. Starving the body of calories and nutrients shuts its metabolism down. As a health coach, weight loss specialist, and personal trainer, I have had many clients who truly believe the only way to lose weight is to eat no more than 1,200 calories a day and exercise like a fanatic. Some clients lost weight, but unfortunately deprived themselves of certain food groups that are necessary for the body to function properly. Thus, when they went off the diet, they gained back the weight they lost and more. This is typical. Water weight comes off first, then fat loss over time. If you rush to lose weight, measure out your food, and then weigh yourself, you are setting yourself up for failure. The stress on your body mentally and physically takes a toll and your cortisol levels start to rise, thus stopping you from losing weight. In addition, when you overexercise, you put undo stress on your body and burn calories temporarily. When you exercise, you actually need to eat more to make up for lost fluids and nutrients. Otherwise, you burn the calories, and anything else you eat later in the day—without the right amount of nutrients and healthy fats—gets stored back in the body as body fat. This is why most women don't see much of a change on the scale when they go on a diet, especially after the first month; they hit a plateau.

One of the things I teach in my weight loss classes is how to eat for health and how to choose the correct foods for each individual's body. It's about bio-individuality. Everyone's body acts and reacts differently to foods, stress, environment, exercise, etc. I discuss what real, whole clean foods are, and how to incorporate them into daily life. I also discuss how to make small, lasting changes. Lifestyle changes become lasting over time. They can't be rushed, or else you tend to go back to old patterns of eating as a comfort. Think of it as how a baby first crawls before it walks. It is the same principle. Relearning how to eat properly for your body is key. It takes time, dedication, and patience. Hiring a health coach or relying on a partner, friend, or other support system to track your progress is important for follow-through.

For weight loss, people tend to forget that our bodies are made up of approximately two-thirds water. When we don't drink enough water each day (rule of thumb: slowly work your way up to drinking half your weight in ounces), we get dehydrated. Then our bodies tend to trick our brains into thinking we're hungry when actually we are dehydrated! So, before you grab junk food, etc., reach for a glass of water, herbal tea, or broth. Then wait 20 minutes, and if you still feel hungry, choose mindfully. I also don't think people realize that digestion begins in the mouth, so it's important to chew slowly rather than rushing. Take some deep breaths before you put anything in your mouth and be calm. Rushing around all day and then eating in a rush serves no purpose for you or your body. As you begin to realize that this is a common pattern for you, you can slowly start to eat more consciously. Don't eat while watching TV or reading, as we tend to eat more and mindlessly when we focus on something else. Focus on you and what is really going on for you. Food can nourish us, but it can also hinder us if we do not eat consciously.

Learning to love yourself deeply takes time, commitment, and patience. It took my grandmother's passing a few years ago for this to really hit me. She always told me to love myself, and I often questioned what that really meant. She wanted me to figure it out for myself, and I'm glad she did. I always thought I loved myself on some level, but not to the extent of what my grandmother meant. You want to love yourself, not out of ego or selfishness, but out of true, deep caring. This could take a few years, or even decades, for some people. There is no time frame here. It is a life-long lesson for all of us. Learn to hear that inner voice that speaks to you, the one you want to get rid of or ignore so often. Getting in touch with that part of us that really wants to love and nourish ourselves is about finding that deep connection within. If you want to feel complete and fulfilled, make the time and commit to getting there.

Chapter 5

Dining Out

Dining out can be relaxing or stressful. You can make it more relaxing by planning ahead. Sometimes you have no choice but to eat out. Perhaps you are working late, traveling, going out with friends, running around with the kids, or maybe you don't enjoy cooking. Whatever the reason, it is important to plan ahead, if possible. Scout out a few places in the area, and select the best and healthiest places for dining out. Look at the menu choices and decide which are the healthiest options.

Keep in mind the goals you have set for yourself. If one of them is to lose weight, then remember that. If you have time to eat a healthy snack beforehand, I highly recommend this. It will help you to be less hungry and to avoid making unhealthy choices at the restaurant. Also, if you are on a tight budget, it is a great way to save money as well as calories! Below is a list of foods that I recommend you avoid or eat in moderation, as well as a list of foods to include in your meal, or ask for.

What to Avoid or Limit

1. *The Bread Basket:* Although it is quite tempting, it fills you up with refined carbs that fill you up with empty calories and add to your waistline. Tell the waiter/waitress beforehand to bring a salad instead of bread.

2. *Salad Dressings:* They are loaded with sugar, sodium, bad fats, preservatives, and chemicals. In finer restaurants, opt for the house dressing or ask for olive oil and vinegar or a slice of lemon. If these are not options, it is best to get vinaigrette dressings rather than ones with cheese or creamy dressings.

3. *Fried Foods:* These include french fries, fried vegetables, tempura, fried appetizers—basically anything greasy. This is probably the most important category to avoid because fried foods cause inflammation and increase the chance of digestive issues, as well as other health concerns down the road. Look for steamed, poached, broiled, or grilled instead.

4. *Heavy Sauces:* Avoid sauces such as alfredo, vodka sauce, heavy cream sauces, and soups. More often than not, they are loaded with too much sodium and

bad fats. Just the sauce alone can include more than a day's supply of fat and sodium! Opt for natural juice or broth in dishes.

5. *Cheese:* Although cheese is yummy and filling, it can add 200 calories or more to a dish. Go easy on the cheese, please!

6. *Alcohol:* Consider that each glass (8 oz.) is at least 100 calories, and that is for just wine or beer! Mixed drinks are loaded with sugar and artificial ingredients and can be 200 calories or more just for one drink. Limit yourself to one or two drinks and consider having the drink for dessert instead! Remember also that drinking alcohol dehydrates the body, so drink water beforehand and afterwards.

7. *Dessert:* It is best to skip dessert if you can. It's easy to overeat when dining out. If you're really craving some dessert, either share or be mindful of what you choose. Avoid high-calorie, high-fat, and high-sugar options.

What to Include and Ask For

1. *Water:* Ask for water or carbonated water with a slice of lemon or lime. Drinking water first fills you up a bit and may help you avoid making poor menu choices.

2. *Condiments:* If available at the restaurant, eat the olives, bean salad, coleslaw, (avoid some of the mayonnaise by draining it off a bit), or pickle (1) instead of the bread.

3. *Appetizers:* If no condiments are offered and you feel very hungry, sharing an appetizer is the way to go. Remember, avoid greasy fried foods. Opt for steamed and preferably something with vegetables in it. A salad is the best appetizer with dressing on the side, preferably oil/vinegar or lemon. Edamame is also a good choice, as well as hummus with vegetable crudité. If you are having soup, opt for broths, vegetable soups, or bean soups. Bear in mind that soups tend to be high in sodium. It is best not to order protein as an appetizer if you are already ordering that as your main dish. People eat way too much animal protein, especially when dining out.

4. *Main Meal:* Choose dishes that are baked, poached, grilled, and cooked in natural juices. Ask for sauces on the side and use sparingly if at all. Limit protein portion size to 6–8 oz. Bring home the rest for leftovers!

5. **Vegetables:** Include vegetables, either steamed or sautéed lightly in olive oil or butter. Ask your waiter or the chef to do this; otherwise, they cook in vegetable oils, which are known to cause inflammation. Order a baked sweet potato or spaghetti squash, as well, if offered. Fill your plate with more vegetables than protein.

I thought it would be helpful to research some of the most popular healthier fast food chain restaurants. I selected 10. Based on the publicly available nutritional data provided by each restaurant, I picked two choices per meal that were comprised, in my opinion, of the least amount of sodium, unhealthy fats, sugar, and other ingredients. (*Note:* some of the restaurants did not list all of the ingredients.) I decided to add to the chart healthier snack and dessert options for those I know who cannot seem to resist when dining out. If you can skip the dessert, yes, it would be better. If you cannot, then I say "go for it" indulge a little and without guilt! (*Note:* If you tend to eat out more than once or twice a week, and have a goal to lose weight, then having dessert might not be in your best interest.) Think of what your goals are first and make the best choices from there. Remember to refer to page 27 and 28 for what to avoid or limit when dining out, and to the chart below as a reference guide before you place your order.

Once you get in the habit of ordering healthier foods, you will notice how much better you feel! You can still eat out and enjoy your food. Making healthier choices is getting easier these days. Just be on the lookout for hidden ingredients. Have fun and enjoy!

Healthier Fast Food Restaurant Chains	Breakfast	Lunch	Dinner	Snacks	Dessert
Au Bon Pain Offers petit plates, healthy snack options, and is allergy friendly.	2 eggs on multi-grain bread/ flatbread *or* scrambled eggs or oatmeal	Veggie & hummus wrap *or* southwest chicken salad	Roasted chicken & thyme entrée *or* 1/2 veggie soup & 1/2 tuna salad sandwich	Petite plate— chicken/ chick pea & tomato salad *or* Mediterranean power pack	Fruit cup *or* mixed nuts
Bare Burger (my favorite) Offers organic dairy & vegetables, pasture-raised & antibiotic-free meats. Vegetarian and allergy friendly.	Not offered	Natural antibiotic-free turkey burger wrapped in gluten free bun or a collard green (original!)	Grass-fed beef burger with veggies and baby kale salad	Sweet potato fries *or* wasabi carrot slaw	Flourless chocolate cake *or* vegan carrot cake
Boston Market Offers healthier choice menu with several options for chicken, turkey, and fresh vegetables.	Not offered	Southwest Santa Fe salad *or* Mediterranean chicken carver sandwich	Three-piece rotisserie chicken (skinless) *or* reg. turkey breast & steamed vegetables or green beans Squash or sweet potato casserole	Chicken noodle soup *or* Caesar salad	Cinnamon apples *or* apple pie
California Pizza Kitchen Offers many salad options, small plates, vegetarian and allergy friendly.	Not offered	Quinoa & arugula salad *or* roasted veggie half with chicken	Cedar plank salmon *or* grilled chicken chimichurri	Dakota smashed pea & barley cup *or* asparagus & arugula salad	Belgian chocolate soufflé cake *or* Tiramisu. Share to save on calories & sugar
Cheesecake Factory Offers many healthy salads, small plates, and lower-calorie options.	Plain omelet or create an omelet with onions, mushrooms, spinach, peppers	Chinese chicken salad *or* simply grilled salmon with a side of veggies	Chicken piccata *or* grilled turkey burger with a side of veggies	Edamame *or* skinnylicious grilled artichoke	Fresh strawberries or plain *or* pumpkin cheesecake slice to share

Healthier Fast Food Restaurant Chains	Breakfast	Lunch	Dinner	Snacks	Dessert
Chipotle Mexican Grill Serves naturally raised meats & dairy and some organic foods, as well.	Not offered	Salad with chicken & fajita veggies *or* corn tortilla with pinto beans, brown rice, cheese, & lettuce	Burrito bowl— chicken *or* steak with brown rice, beans & fajita veggies	Chips & guacamole *or* chips & roasted chili-corn salsa	Same as snacks
Così Offers many healthy options and all natural chicken.	Oatmeal with fresh strawberries or raisins *or* multigrain flatbread with plain or veggie cream cheese	Hummus & veggie sandwich w/ side salad *or* grilled chicken salad & add own toppings: peppers, tomatoes, sweet potato, cucumbers, corn & black bean mix, avocado	Adobe chicken with avocado bowl and side baby kale salad *or* turkey light sandwich w/ side salad	Bag of carrots *or* side of turkey chili *or* side of chicken noodle soup or tomato basil	Cranberry orange or blueberry scone
Panera Bread Offers many healthy options and antibiotic-free chicken and turkey.	Power almond quinoa oatmeal *or* avocado, egg white & spinach breakfast power sandwich	Mediterranean chicken flatbread (1) sandwich *or* classic with chicken salad	Roasted turkey & avocado on sourdough *or* Asian sesame chicken salad	Power chicken hummus bowl *or* cup low-fat vegetarian garden veg. soup with pesto	Apple or 1 bag baked crisps *or* shortbread cookie (1) *or* petite chocolate chipper (1)
Romano's Macaroni Grill Offers salads and lite menu options.	Not offered	Lentil soup w/ side salad *or* Carmela's chicken pasta *or* mushroom ravioli *or* pollo caprese	Mediterranean branzino fish *or* chicken marsala w/ side greens or Caesar salad	Goat cheese peppadew peppers *or* stuffed mushrooms	Sorbet or gelato
Ruby Tuesday's Offers Fit & Trim selections and several fresh vegetable sides.	Not offered	Fit & Trim Petite Plate sliced sirloin with zucchini, broccoli, and/or spaghetti squash *or* grilled chicken salad	Grilled salmon *or* hickory bourbon chicken with zucchini, broccoli, and/or spaghetti squash	Sweet potato fries *or* 6 cheese & tomato flatbread *or* bbq chicken flatbread *or* Thai spring rolls	Carrot cake cupcake *or* chocolate chip cookie (1) *or* 1 white chocolate macadamia nut cookie

Chapter 6

Making Simple, Easy Meals at Home

Plan Ahead

Whether you are a cook or just a beginner, if you can find no time in your typical day for meal planning, this is a good way to start. Put aside one hour on the weekend to plan a menu and shopping list for the week.

1. *Calendar.* Have a separate calendar with plenty of room to write in just for meal planning. Mark down when you will shop, when you will prep, and when you will cook. If plans change, have a backup of where you will go to eat (see Chapter 5, Dining Out).

2. *Menu.* On a separate piece of paper (or better yet, use your computer to save for future reference), write down a menu for the week. Over time, you can make a few different weekly menus to refer to so you don't get bored eating the same things over and over again.

   • Include family/kids when planning meals to make it easier and fun!
   • Make menus simple, not complicated (see sample menu below).

3. *Shopping and Shopping List.* Try to shop only one day a week to save time and money. If you need more produce and other missed items, then pick another day during the week, such as a Wednesday. It's always best to be ahead of yourself and your meals, for you and your family, rather than fall behind and make poor choices. Make a shopping list of all items for that week as best as possible. Include all staples.

   • Write down items needed for that week's meals (check what staples you have to avoid duplication).

   • To make things easier, organize the list by section in the store, such as produce, refrigerator/frozen foods, meats, staples, etc. This will save time while shopping.

- Keep a running list of staples/items, and when you run out of something, put it on the list again

- Enlist your family to help, no matter how young. Supermarkets today are kid friendly, with shopping carts that have cars connected to them. Have your kids search for items. Make it like a treasure hunt. Come up with healthy snacks for them to search for rather than the usual boxed or packaged snacks. It's best to stick to your shopping list, especially with kids, so you don't end up buying unnecessary items, such as junk food.

- Buy pre-cut vegetables to save time and effort if that holds you back from cooking.

- Eat organic when you can: Avoiding pesticides and other chemicals on produce is important for you and your family. *The Environmental Working Group's 2015 (EWG) Dirty Dozen-Plus List of non-organic produce that is important to avoid includes the following:*

  1. Apple
  2. Strawberries
  3. Grapes
  4. Celery
  5. Peaches
  6. Spinach
  7. Sweet Bell Peppers
  8. Nectarines (Imported)
  9. Cucumbers
  10. Cherry Tomatoes
  11. Snap Peas (Imported)
  12. Potatoes
  + Hot Peppers
  + Kale/Collard Greens

- *Here is the List of the Clean 15 foods according to EWG that are lowest in pesticides.* If you cannot find or afford organic, just the items on this list would be acceptable for non-organic, as well.

  1. Avocados
  2. Sweet Corn (I recommend organic and non-GMO)
  3. Pineapples
  4. Cabbage
  5. Sweet Peas (Frozen)
  6. Onions
  7. Asparagus
  8. Mangoes
  9. Papayas
  10. Kiwi
  11. Eggplant
  12. Grapefruit
  13. Cantaloupe
  14. Cauliflower
  15. Sweet Potatoes

4. *Preparation*

- Wash and chop most vegetables in advance, such as carrots, celery, cabbage, broccoli, cauliflower, kale, onions, etc., or buy pre-cut vegetables to save time and effort if it holds you back from cooking. Softer vegetables such as tomatoes, cucumbers, peppers, and lettuce should not be chopped in advance, as they will spoil faster and bruise or wilt.

- Prepare extra food for leftovers. Leftovers are great for lunch and dinner, and they save you from having to cook daily. Make a large vegetable dish, bean dish, or grain dish to add to other foods for variety over the course of a few days.

- Cook more in advance and freeze in portions. This will save you time and effort for the following week or two.

For convenience, I have included a shopping list and sample menu charts for the beginner and for the more advanced cook. I made several suggestions for each meal, including a healthy snack, great for midday slumps or evening snacks. I thought out each menu carefully and hope you enjoy the suggestions. As a bonus, you might actually lose weight by following the menus!

I also have included some simple recipes that take less than 30 minutes to make for the beginner cook, and other simple recipes that might take a bit longer for the more advanced cook or someone who has a bit more time on their hands. See shopping lists, menus, and recipes on the next few pages.

Sample Menu for the Beginner Cook

Breakfast	Lunch	Healthy Snack	Dinner
Hard-boiled eggs	Fresh turkey on a whole grain wrap or lettuce wrap with tomato and cucumber sliced thin	Cauliflower soup (see recipe)	Lentils with quinoa (see recipes) Steamed mixed vegetables
Oatmeal—rolled oats or steel cut Add cinnamon and a small amount of dried fruit or diced apples	Natural peanut butter or almond butter on whole grain bread Cut up cucumbers & baby carrots	Sweet potato fries (see recipe section)	Store-bought, free-range or organic rotis-serie chicken (save bones for bone broth recipe) String beans
Laura's green smoothie (see recipe section)	Roasted chicken cut up with romaine lettuce and 4 other veggies of choice	Cut-up veggies and hummus	Turkey burger, steamed broccoli, and salad
Chicken or turkey breakfast sausage and 1 slice of 100% whole grain bread with a little butter, natural peanut or almond butter	Veggie burger with steamed string beans, broccoli, or salad	Kale chips (see recipe)	Bone broth (see recipe) with leftover diced rotis-serie chicken. Add carrots, celery, and onion to broth & spinach at end. Can add leftover quinoa or brown rice to broth
Scrambled eggs, whole grain bread with butter	Hummus, lettuce, spinach, tomato, avocado, sprouts in a whole grain or rice wrap	Apple slices with natural peanut or almond butter	Baked fresh salmon fillet Steamed brown rice, roasted zucchini & asparagus spears

Sample Menu for the More Advanced Cook

Breakfast	Lunch	Healthy Snack	Dinner
Protein shake Milk or almond milk with sprouted rice protein powder, frozen 1/2 banana, and/or berries, & spinach. Can add soaked nuts/seeds or flax meal or chia seeds, coconut and/or natural cocoa powder, Stevia drops to sweeten or 1 tsp. raw honey. Blend all together.	Tuna or salmon salad mixed with mashed avocado instead of mayo, or try mustard with whole grain bread or on a bed of lettuce with 4 other veggies	Roasted root vegetables (see advanced recipe section)	Grilled chicken with mixed vegetables and salad
Quinoa Add cinnamon and a small amount of dried fruit or diced apples. Add milk if desired.	Salad made with lettuce, spinach, cucumber, chickpeas, or black beans, avocado topped with some roasted root veggies	Trail mix Mix of raw almonds, walnuts, pumpkin and/or sunflower seeds (1/8-1/4 cup total) plus 1/4 cup of unsweetened coconut flakes, raisins, natural semi-sweet chocolate chips	Laura's slow cooker chicken with vegetables (see advanced recipe section) Mixed greens salad
Laura's super nutritious green smoothie (see advanced recipe section)	Grilled chicken strips with romaine lettuce, cucumbers, peppers, tomatoes, radishes, avocado	Celery sticks with natural peanut or almond butter	Ground turkey or ground (grass-fed) beef meatballs w/spaghetti squash (see recipe) and steamed green beans
Natural, (nitrate free) chicken or turkey breakfast sausage and 1 slice of 100% whole grain bread with a little butter or natural peanut or almond butter	Lean ground turkey or beef in a taco shell with shredded lettuce, tomato, diced cucumber, sprouts, slice of avocado	Marv's mock chopped liver pate (see advanced recipe) w/ rice crackers or cut-up veggies	Homemade chicken soup with bone broth (see advanced recipe)
Vegetable omelet with onions, spinach, broccoli, peppers, etc.	Quinoa salad (see advanced recipe section)	Chocolate kale chips (see advanced recipe)	Baked fresh salmon fillet Steamed brown rice, roasted zucchini & asparagus spears

Shopping List for Beginner Recipes

Vegetables
Cauliflower
Sweet Potatoes (3–4 long potatoes)
Romaine Lettuce
Spinach
Carrots (bag)
Cucumber (1)
Celery
Onion (1 large)

Fruit
Apple (1) or Banana (1) and/or 1/2 cup Berries (for green smoothie)

Grains/Beans
Quinoa
Lentils (green)

Oil/Butter
Unrefined Coconut Butter, Butter or Ghee (clarified butter)

Condiments/Spices
Non-Irradiated Cinnamon
Chia Seeds or Ground Flax Meal
Sea Salt or Celtic Sea Salt
Stevia—liquid drops

Chicken Bones
Save from leftover cooked chicken or purchase bones or
box of low-sodium chicken or vegetable broth

Shopping List for More Advanced Recipes

Vegetables
Parsley (bunch)
Kale (1–2 bunches)
Romaine Lettuce
Spinach
Carrots (bunch)
Cucumber (1)
Celery
Onions (3)
4 Cloves Garlic (minced)
Sweet Potatoes or Winter Squash
(1-1/2 pounds)
3 lb. Spaghetti Squash
1–2 Rutabagas
2 Parsnips
2 Turnips

Fruit
Apple (1) or Banana (1) and/or
1/2 cup Berries (for green smoothie)

Grains/Beans
Quinoa
Lentils (green)

Oil/Butter/Eggs
Unrefined Coconut Butter, Butter or
Ghee (clarified butter)* (organic preferred)
First Cold Pressed Extra Virgin Olive Oil
6 eggs

* You can find these at many better
supermarkets, health food stores,
farmers markets, and online.

Condiments/Spices
Onion Powder
Garlic Powder
Thyme
Black Pepper
Italian Seasoning
Sea Salt or Celtic Sea Salt
Red Pepper (crushed) (optional)
1 28-ounce can no-salt-added
Crushed Tomatoes
Natural Cocoa Powder
Stevia—liquid drops
Natural Cinnamon (non-irradiated is best)
Raw Honey or 100% Maple Syrup
Vanilla Extract (avoid corn syrup)

Nuts/Seeds
Chia Seeds or Ground Flax Meal
(you can find these in better
supermarkets and in health food stores)
4 oz. Raw Cashews or small jar
Raw Cashew or Almond Butter
4 oz. Raw Walnuts (ground)

Meats/Bones
Chicken Bones
(Save from leftover cooked chicken or
purchase bones or box of low-sodium
chicken or vegetable broth)
Cooked cut-up chicken for soup
1 pound ground turkey for meatballs

All About Quinoa

Quinoa (pronounced "keen-wah") is a seed from Peru. Native people of the Andes have used Quinoa in cooking for over 5,000 years. It is known as the "mother grain." It is eaten as one would eat rice or any other grain. However, it is not a true grain. Quinoa comes from the goosefoot family of plants, which includes spinach, beets, and Swiss chard. The leaves of quinoa can be eaten just like spinach. It is considered a complete protein, containing an almost perfect balance of all 8 essential amino acids, unlike any true grain. It is exceptionally high in lysine, methionine, and cysteine, which are typically low in other grains. One cup has 8.14 grams of protein. Quinoa also contains more iron than other grains, as well as high levels of potassium, riboflavin, B6, niacin and thiamin. It is also a good source of magnesium, zinc copper, manganese, and fiber.

Quinoa has a light, delicious taste, is easy to digest, and contains no gluten. You can find it in health food stores and in some larger supermarkets. It is either boxed in the grain section in supermarkets or found in the bulk section. If you buy it in bulk, store the grain in a tightly closed container in a cool, dry place.

Simple Recipes for Beginner Cooks

Simple Quinoa

Ingredients

1 cup quinoa
2 cups water
Sea salt to taste

Rinse quinoa thoroughly in a fine strainer until the water runs clear; drain well. This will remove any bitter, powdery residue.

For a delicious, roasted flavor, toast the grain in a dry skillet for 5 minutes before cooking.

To cook, use two parts water to one part dry quinoa. Combine water and quinoa in a medium saucepan, bring to boil. Add a dash of sea salt when cooking. Reduce heat to a simmer, cover and cook for another 15 minutes or until the grains are translucent and the germ has spiraled out from each grain. Season with sea salt and butter, ghee, or olive oil at the end of cooking.

For breakfast. Reheat leftover quinoa, and have it instead of oatmeal with milk (cow, rice, soy, or almond), cinnamon, steamed fruit or raisins and slivers of almonds, sunflower seeds, or pumpkin seeds.

For Lunch or Dinner

Quinoa Pilaf

Ingredients

1 cup quinoa—rinsed and drained
2 cups water or low-sodium chicken or vegetable broth for added flavor
1/2 cup chopped onion

Directions

Sauté chopped onion in olive oil on low to medium heat. Add toasted quinoa (as described above) and water.

Simmer covered with a lid for 15 minutes. After pilaf is cooked, stir in other ingredients to your liking, such as toasted nuts, dried fruit, shredded greens, diced vegetables, and/or fresh herbs.

Lentils

Lentils are a good source of protein and fiber. They also contain many vitamins and minerals and can help reduce heart disease and cancer.

Ingredients

2 cups dried green lentils (soaked overnight)
6–7 cups water
1 small onion, cut up
1 carrot, quartered
2 celery stalks with leaves, quartered
1 clove garlic, crushed (optional)
Kombu or kelp (optional)
Sea salt to taste

Directions

Soak lentils overnight with a piece of kombu or seaweed. This helps with digestion, adds flavor and many nutrients, and speeds up the cooking time.

Rinse and drain lentils and kombu. Place kombu in the bottom of a pot. Place rinsed lentils in pot with water, onion, carrot, celery, and garlic.

Bring to a boil, cover, and simmer until the lentils are tender, about 1 hour. Season with sea salt.

Makes approximately 2 quarts of lentils.

Easy Bone Broth

Buy a rotisserie chicken (preferably a free range, all-natural chicken) and debone it. Save the meat for soup, salads, and other dishes.

Reserve the bones and drippings or gelatin on the bottom of the container from two or more chickens. Cut the already soft bones in half or coarse pieces. This will open up the marrow from the bones, which will add nutrients to the broth. You can also freeze the bones to make the broth at a later date—a great way to save time and money.

Ingredients

Chicken bones (cut up) from 2 or more chickens
4 quarts cold water (filtered or spring water is preferred)
2 tablespoons apple cider vinegar or fresh lemon
1 large onion, coarsely chopped
2 carrots, peeled and coarsely chopped
3 celery stalks, coarsely chopped
1 bunch parsley
Sea salt (after cooking)

Directions

Place the cut-up bones, drippings, water, and vegetables (with the exception of the parsley) in a large stock pot or slow cooker. Add the vinegar or lemon and let sit for 30 minutes to 1 hour. This helps the minerals leach out of the bones and into the broth.

Bring to a boil if cooking in a pot, or put on high if using a slow cooker, for the first 3–4 hours, then simmer for 6–24 hours.

During the last 10 minutes of cooking, add a bunch of parsley for added minerals and flavor.

Add sea salt to taste.

Remove the bones with a slotted spoon and strain broth into another pot. Store up to 7 days in fridge or freeze in mason jars up to 6 months. Use broth for soups or stews, or drink throughout the day instead of water, coffee, or tea. It's much healthier, and your body will reap the benefits!

Recipe Adapted from *Nourishing Traditions*

Laura's Cauliflower Soup (or Blended "Mock" Potatoes)

This is quite simple to make and a healthier substitute for white potatoes. You might even get your kids to like it!

Ingredients

1 head cauliflower, cut into pieces
1/4 cup butter or unrefined coconut oil
Sea salt to taste
For making soup, add 3–4 cups low-sodium vegetable or chicken broth

Directions

Steam the cauliflower until tender. Reserve the water from the pot.
Take the cauliflower and blend in a blender until it is pureed. Add the butter or coconut oil (adds a nice flavor and good for you, too) and sea salt. Blend all together. Reheat if necessary and add the reserved water.

Cauliflower soup: Add the blended cauliflower mixture to another pot with vegetable or chicken broth. Reheat and serve.

For variations, add to blended mixture:
Grated daikon radish
Zucchini squash (peeled)
Sautéed onions or leeks (white part)

Laura's Baked Sweet Potato Fries

A great snack for you and your kids! The cinnamon brings out the natural sweetness of the sweet potatoes.

Ingredients

3–4 long sweet potatoes
1–2 tablespoons raw coconut oil (note: oil is solid in cold weather, liquid in warm)
1–2 teaspoons cinnamon

Directions:

Pre-heat oven to 375 degrees F.
Peel, wash, and cut potatoes into sticks or half moon shapes.
Place on a large cookie sheet or baking dish.
Add coconut oil & cinnamon. Mix well to coat each vegetable lightly with oil and cinnamon.

Bake uncovered for 35–45 minutes until vegetables are tender and golden brown, checking every 10 minutes to stir and make sure veggies are not sticking.

Roasted Kale with Sea Salt

Ingredients

4 cups firmly packed kale
1–2 tablespoons extra virgin olive oil or unrefined coconut oil
(better flavor and for high heat)
1 teaspoon good-quality sea salt

Directions

Preheat oven to 375 degrees F.
Wash and trim the kale: Peel off the tough stems by folding the kale leaves in half like a book and stripping the stems off. Toss with extra virgin olive oil. Roast for five minutes. Turn kale over. Roast another 5–10 minutes, depending on your oven, until kale turns brown and becomes paper thin and brittle. Be sure to watch kale, as it can burn easily.
Remove from oven and sprinkle with sea salt. Serve immediately.

Yes, your kids will learn to love this snack, too!

Laura's Super Nutritious Green Smoothie

Ingredients

4–6 romaine lettuce leaves
1 peeled carrot, cut up
1/2–1 cup spinach leaves
1/4 of a cucumber (peeled)
1/2 to 1 small apple, peeled & cut up, or 1/2 banana frozen, or 1/2 cup berries
1–2 tablespoons ground flax meal or soaked chia seeds
1/2–3/4 cup water, milk, unsweetened almond milk, or coconut milk
Stevia drops (5–7 drops) for added sweetness or 1 tsp raw honey

Directions

It is best to use organic produce whenever possible. Feel free to add other veggies for variety and taste.

Wash, cut up, and add all vegetables, apple or other fruit, ground flax meal or soaked chia seeds, and water or milk into a high-powered blender. Blend until smooth.

Add Stevia drops (no more than 5–7 drops; it's 100 times sweeter than sugar!) or honey. You can also add vanilla, natural cocoa powder, or natural protein powder for added flavor.

Eat/drink slowly by chewing well and let your taste buds get used to something new and good for you! Your body will reap the benefits! Change takes time, so your taste buds will need time to get used to the smoothie. Some people choose to take a digestive enzyme with the smoothie to make digestion easier. Enjoy!

Recipes for Advanced Cooks

Marv's Mock Chopped Liver

Ingredients

1 lb. frozen peas, thawed and cooked well until soft or 15-1/2 oz. can sweet peas (drained)
1 cup finely ground walnuts (approximately a 4-oz. bag of already-ground walnuts)
4 hard-boiled eggs
1 to 1-1/2 large onions, diced and sautéed in a little olive oil

Directions

Blend all (except for approximately 2 tablespoons of the sautéed onion) in a food processor. Add salt/pepper. Add the rest of the sautéed onions to the mix and refrigerate.

Recipe given by my late cousin Marv.

Laura's Chicken Soup

Ingredients

4 quarts of pre-made bone broth or two boxes of low-sodium bone broth, chicken broth, or vegetable broth

Add

Celtic sea salt to taste
Black pepper to taste (optional)
1 small onion, chopped
4 carrots, sliced
3 celery ribs, chopped
2 parsnips, sliced
1 or 2 turnips, coarsely chopped
Parsley, handful
1 small sweet potato cut in large chunks (if you want sweeter soup)
Pieces of cooked chicken

Simmer broth with additional vegetables for 1 hour. Add cooked chicken for last 15 minutes until warm, and serve.

(A variation of my mother's and grandmother's soup)

Quinoa Salad

Ingredients

1 cup quinoa, dry
2 cups water
1 finely chopped red bell pepper
1/2 cucumber, diced
1 bunch finely diced scallions (mainly white part)
1/4 cup finely diced cilantro or parsley
1–1 1/2 lemons or limes, squeezed
2 tablespoons sesame oil
2 tablespoons raw honey (optional)
Sea salt to taste

Optional
Add garbanzo beans or other beans for added nutrition

Directions

Rinse quinoa. Bring water, sea salt, and quinoa to a boil, then reduce to a simmer and cover. Cook for 15 minutes. Uncover, fluff, and cool immediately. Add sesame oil, honey, lime or lemon juice, and cilantro or parsley. Stir in vegetables until quinoa is coated evenly. Great as a side dish or for lunch.

Laura's Slow Cooker Chicken and Vegetables

Ingredients

1/2–1 teaspoon sea salt
1 teaspoon onion powder
1 teaspoon thyme
1/2 teaspoon garlic powder
1/4 teaspoon black pepper
1 large onion
1 lb. winter squash or sweet potato cut into large chunks
1 or 2 large rutabagas cut into large chunks
1 large chicken or cut-up parts (dark meat is best)

Directions

Combine the dried spices in a small bowl.

Loosely chop the onion and place it in the bottom of the slow cooker. Add vegetables.

Remove any giblets from the chicken and then rub the spice mixture all over. You can even put some of the spices inside the cavity and under the skin covering the breasts.

Put prepared chicken on top of the onions and vegetables in the slow cooker, cover it, and turn it to high. There is no need to add any liquid.

Cook for about 4 hours on high (for a 3- to 4-pound chicken) or on low for about 5–6 hours, until the chicken is falling off the bone.

Spaghetti Squash & Meatballs

Ingredients

1 3-pound spaghetti squash
1/4–1/2 cup water
2 tablespoons extra virgin olive oil, divided
1/2 cup chopped fresh parsley, divided
1-1/4 teaspoons Italian seasoning, divided
1/2 teaspoon onion powder
1/2 teaspoon sea salt, divided
1/2 teaspoon freshly ground pepper
1 pound ground turkey or beef
4 cloves garlic, minced
1 28-ounce can no-salt-added crushed tomatoes
1/4–1/2 tsp crushed red pepper (optional)

Directions

Halve squash lengthwise and scoop out the seeds. Place face down in a baking dish; add approximately 1/2 cup water to bottom of dish. Bake in oven at 375 degrees F for about 45 minutes. (This step can be done the day before.)

Heat 1 tablespoon of oil in a large skillet over medium heat. Scrape the squash flesh into the skillet and cook, stirring occasionally, until the moisture is evaporated and the squash is beginning to brown, 5–10 minutes. Stir in 1/4 cup parsley. Remove from heat and let stand.

Meanwhile, combine the remaining 1/4 cup parsley, 1/2 teaspoon Italian seasoning, onion powder, 1/4 teaspoon salt and pepper in a medium bowl. Add turkey or beef; gently mix to combine (do not over-mix). Using about 2 tablespoons for each one, form into 12 meatballs.

Heat the remaining 1 tablespoon oil in a large skillet over medium heat. Add the meatballs, turning occasionally, until browned all over, 4–6 minutes. Push the meatballs to the side of the pan; add garlic and cook, stirring, for 1 minute.

Add tomatoes, crushed red pepper to taste, the remaining 3/4 teaspoon Italian seasoning, and 1/4 teaspoon salt; stir to coat the meatballs. Bring to a simmer, cover and cook, stirring occasionally, until the meatballs are cooked through, 10–12 minutes.

Serve the sauce and meatballs over the squash.

Adapted from "Recipe: Spaghetti Squash & Meatballs." *Eating Well* Jan.–Feb. 2015: 32.

Laura's Super Nutritious Green Smoothie

Ingredients

4–6 romaine lettuce leaves
1 stalk celery, cut up
1 peeled carrot, cut up
Handful of fresh parsley, stems removed (adds super nutrition*)
2–3 kale leaves (adds super nutrition*)
1/2–1 cup spinach leaves
1/4 of a cucumber (peeled)
1/2 to 1 small apple, peeled and cut up, or 1/2 banana frozen, or 1/2 cup berries
1–2 tablespoons ground flax meal or soaked chia seeds
1/2–3/4 cup water, milk, unsweetened almond milk, or coconut milk
Stevia drops (5–7 drops) for added sweetness, or 1 tsp. raw honey

It is best to use organic produce whenever possible. Feel free to add other veggies for variety and taste.

Directions

Wash, cut up, and add all vegetables, apple or other fruit, ground flax meal or soaked chia seeds, and water or milk into a high-powered blender. Blend until smooth.

Add stevia drops (no more than 5–7 drops; it's 100 times sweeter than sugar!) or honey. You can also add vanilla, natural cocoa powder, or natural protein powder for added flavor.

Eat/drink slowly by chewing well and let your taste buds get used to something new and good for you! Your body will reap the benefits!

Change takes time, so your taste buds will need time to get used to the smoothie. Some people choose to take a digestive enzyme with the smoothie to make digestion easier. Enjoy!

Note: parsley and kale are super nutritious; add only one at first to acquire the taste.

Roasted Root Vegetables

Ingredients

1 medium winter squash
2 parsnips
2 carrots
1 large rutabaga
1 daikon radish
Extra virgin olive oil or raw unrefined coconut oil
Salt and pepper
Herbs like: rosemary, thyme, or sage (fresh, if possible) or for a sweeter
  taste, add cinnamon

Directions

Pre-heat oven to 375 degrees F.

Wash and chop all vegetables into large bite-sized pieces.
Place in a large baking dish with sides.

Drizzle with olive oil or coconut oil; mix well to coat each vegetable lightly with oil.
Sprinkle with salt, pepper, and herbs or cinnamon.

Bake uncovered for 25–35 minutes until vegetables are tender and golden brown, checking every 10 minutes to stir and make sure veggies are not sticking.

Note: Any combination of vegetables will work. Roasting only one kind of vegetable also makes a nice side dish.

Recipe inspired by IIN ©.

Chocolate Kale Chips

Ingredients

1 bunch of kale, washed, big stems removed,
  and kale cut or broken into medium-sized pieces
1/2 cup cashews, soaked, or 1/2 cup raw cashews
  (can substitute raw almond butter or other raw nut butters)
1/2 cup raw honey/maple syrup (one or a combination)
1/3 cup cocoa powder
1 teaspoon vanilla extract
1/2 teaspoon cinnamon

Optional:
1/4 cup coconut flakes (unsweetened)
2 tablespoons unrefined coconut oil

Directions

Soak cashews in water for at least one hour (4–6 hours is ideal). Remove the soaked cashews and add all other ingredients (except the kale) to a high-powered blender. Blend until mixture is smooth enough to make the chocolate (and coconut) coating. Pour this mixture over a bowl of washed, de-stemmed kale leaves and toss to coat.

Transfer coated kale to a parchment-lined cookie sheet and bake at 300 degrees F for about 20 minutes. Flip and bake for another 8–10 minutes. Watch it closely because the honey and/or maple mixture can burn quickly and, with the dark chocolate color, it's hard to tell if they are burning or not. Let your nose and common sense be your guide. Remove crispy chips one by one if necessary.

You could dehydrate these chips, too, but because many people don't have dehydrators, I purposely made these in the oven.

Recipe adapted from AveryCooks.com

Chapter 7

Making Healthy Choices

We have many options when it comes to choosing the foods we eat. The way we eat affects our daily lives. It can affect our relationships, career, self-esteem, self-worth, and overall health. If we are not balanced, then we throw our eating off balance, as well. Our emotions play a big part in what we eat every day. When we are stressed, we tend to eat high-stress foods. These might include comfort foods to comfort our moods. High dairy or meat consumption, fried foods, fast foods, sugar (such as candy), chocolate, ice cream, cookies, cakes, pizza, and pretzels all fit into this category. Slow down a little each day and take some deep breaths. Have a glass of water or cup of herbal tea. Do some exercises, such as pushups, sit-ups, or walking for a change of scenery. All this can help you before you decide to eat out of stress and frustration. Distracting yourself from the stress is key. As you become aware of what you are doing over time, it will help you break the cycle of stress eating. Including healthier choices and foods when under stress or even when calm will benefit your body. You may notice over time that you don't crave the high-stress foods as much as you used to. Cravings tend to diminish when you supply your body with the foods it needs and wants. This may require you to step out of your comfort zone and try a new food. It takes at least three tries to see if you like a particular food, so give some new healthy foods a chance!

If you want to feel good, energized, and vibrant, choose foods wisely on a daily basis. You can cheat once or twice during the week in moderation (for 1 meal and/or 1 dessert) as long as you eat optimally 80% of the time. This will help keep you on track without depriving yourself of the foods and desserts you love. What our bodies truly want (not what we necessarily desire) and require on a daily basis are nourishing foods that are calming to the body. Here are some suggestions:

Low-Stress Foods/Drinks to Include in Your Diet

- *Low-Sodium Broths.* Homemade is best. Avoid canned broths, as they are too high in sodium. Buy boxed low-sodium broths if you don't have homemade.

- *Herbal Teas.* Make sure they are decaffeinated.

- *Filtered or Natural Spring Water.* Avoid plastic bottles if you can. Drink at least 8 cups a day!

- **Clean Protein.** If you eat meat, make sure it is antibiotic free and, if affordable, grass fed (raised on a farm with organic supplemental feed is optimal). Use pastured poultry and wild fish. (Avoid farm-raised fish, which has antibiotics and chemicals added.) Protein should be no more than the size of a deck of cards or the palm of your hand at each meal.

- **Beans/Legumes.** They are high in protein, fiber, vitamins, and minerals. Beans such as aduki are easiest to digest. Pinto, black, kidney, or navy beans are just as good, but harder to digest. Legumes, such as split peas and lentils, are great to include, as well. If using canned beans, find ones that are low in sodium, and rinse them well before using.

- **Green Vegetables.** Choose ones that are low in starch (see list in Chapter 8).

- **Healthy Fats.** Omega-3 fats are very important. Our bodies don't make this fat, so including various sources is essential. This fat helps reduce stress, inflammation, and is good for brain function and for overall health. Also include avocado and Extra Virgin First Cold Pressed Olive Oil (in dark bottle only); organic is preferable (cook on low/medium heat only or use as a salad dressing).

Eat Whole Foods

Just as the name implies, whole foods are in their "whole" natural state, as they come from nature. Vegetables, fruits, unprocessed grains, legumes, and beans are considered whole foods. Note that in order for a grain to be whole, it has to be in its original state. The whole "germ" or grain has to be intact. Grains that state they are quick cooking, cracked, shredded, flaked, or ground into flours are not whole grains. They are processed. The processed grains get absorbed into the body quickly due to the refined process of the grain. An example of this would be a bagel. The ground flour in a bagel is highly processed, even if it is whole wheat flour. It might taste good and fill you up, but it's empty calories with little nutrition, and it can affect your blood sugar as well, since it gets absorbed quickly into your bloodstream. On the other hand, whole grains, such as brown rice, bulgur, buckwheat, quinoa, and millet get absorbed into the body more slowly and do not affect your blood sugar as much.

Whole foods nourish your body with the nutrients that it needs. When you eat whole foods, you are eating more balanced, nutrient-dense foods that contain all or most of your body's daily required vitamins, and they are absorbed into the body more readily than a vitamin supplement.

Choose to incorporate more whole foods into your daily diet. Notice how you feel after eating this way for a few months. You will reap many benefits by doing so!

Bear in mind that Americans eat much more omega-6 fats than omega-3 fats. While the human body needs a balance of omega 3, 6, and 9 fats, it is important to note where we get these fats from. Too many omega-6 fats cause inflammation in the body and are found in most packaged convenience foods, snacks, and fast foods. They might include vegetable oils, such as soybean, corn, cottonseed, safflower, and sunflower oil. It is best to avoid or limit these types of oils in all foods you eat. You can include natural, raw, unprocessed seeds instead, such as raw sunflower seeds and pumpkin seeds. Remember to also avoid trans fats, which include partially hydrogenated oils. In order to get more omega-3 fats in our diet, we must include them through food and supplementation. They are not supplied naturally by the body. They are also known as essential fatty acids, or EFAs. They are essential to the human body, and most Americans don't get nearly enough of omega-3s in their daily diets. Omega-3s help reduce stress and are good for brain function and overall health. Include wild fish, such as wild salmon, sardines, herring, black cod, or a good quality purified fish oil or krill oil. Ground flax meal or flax oil (do not cook with the oil), walnuts, chia seeds, and hemp seeds are also high in omega-3 fats. Other good sources are dark leafy green vegetables, such as kale, collards, spinach, and mustard greens.

Most of us don't eat nearly enough vegetables, but they are so important in order to give us lasting energy throughout the day. Relying on caffeinated drinks and/or sugar is not the best choice for your body in the long run. Start eating at least 2–3 cups of vegetables per day, then increase by a 1/2 cup every month or so until you get up to 6–9 cups of vegetables per day! Yes, you can do it and learn to love vegetables, too! They give you super energy and also help you lose weight as an added bonus!

Here are some suggestions to add to your daily diet:

- 1 cup raw spinach or 2 cups steamed or sautéed
- 1 cup steamed broccoli, cauliflower, or cabbage
- 2 cups mixed leafy green lettuce
- 1 cup zucchini (grilled, roasted, steamed, or you can even make pasta out of it with a spiralizer)
- 6–10 asparagus spears, grilled or steamed

I chose the above for various reasons. They are all mostly green and easy to find. They all have the necessary vitamins, minerals, and fiber. The deep leafy green vegetables have the highest nutritional value and are the most important to eat daily. Just the calcium content alone helps keep your body and bones strong. The greens also have essential fatty acids, something that our bodies do not make on their own. As stated previously, they are the perfect way to stay energized throughout the day. Once you start to eat spinach, broccoli, and mixed greens comfortably, try the nutrient-dense greens, such as collard greens, kale, chard, arugula, and dandelion. Be careful to not overcook, as these greens tend to turn bitter if overcooked.

I encourage you to add other vegetables with various colors, such as white: onions, cucumber, radish; yellow: yellow squash or yellow peppers; orange: sweet potato or winter squash, etc. The more color and variety of vegetables you eat, the better you will feel.

If you really don't like vegetables, start slow and be daring. It takes at least three attempts to try a new food before you say you don't like it. If you're picky about eating vegetables, and I know many adults who are, then try to blend them into a smoothie or have a fresh extracted juice (see recipe section). I can't stress enough how much your body needs the nutrients from the vegetables. When we buy vitamins, our bodies only absorb a small percentage of them. When we eat live, fresh, and preferably organic vegetables, and even buy local, we are getting the vitamins absorbed properly in our bodies.

Food can promote good health or it can take away from our health. The choice is yours.

Chapter 8

Lose Weight Naturally and Without Dieting!

Typically, diet plans don't work in the long run. They might work for a few months, but due to restrictions on the diet, people tend to go back to their old comfortable ways of eating. When you go on a diet, what you are actually losing is mainly water and muscle. In the process of dieting, you might feel even more stressed because you have eliminated a particular food group or groups. Over time, you feel deprivation from the food group you are missing out on. You might even feel more stress from calorie counting, weighing yourself on a scale, and basically starving your body of the daily nutrients it needs for survival. Then, once the weight is lost, you tend to slowly (or quickly) go back to old eating patterns and gain the weight back, this time in the form of fat storage due to slowing down your metabolism each time you diet.

The truth of the matter is there really is no quick, permanent way to lose weight! You must be patient and learn a lifestyle change so that you can slowly learn how to incorporate healthy, nutrient-dense whole foods into your diet. I have been working with many clients through the years on weight loss and lifestyle changes to help guide them toward optimal and long-lasting results. The main obstacle seems to be people getting in their own way. There is a fear of letting go of the old, comfortable ways of eating and letting go of the actual weight on the body. The weight seems to be a comfort to some and a hindrance to others. Beating yourself up daily because you overate or ate too many so-called "bad" foods sets you up for more failure in the long run. I feel there are really no "bad" or "good" foods. Labeling them this way is treating yourself as a child waiting to be punished for eating incorrectly. It is much better to think of food as nourishment. When we don't eat nourishing foods, we might not feel well physically or mentally, so re-learning how to eat better for "ourselves" is important here. Each person is unique, and our bodies are unique. One food might be good for one person, but not for another.

Here are a few tips on how to start losing weight naturally:

1. *Eat breakfast.* Even if you're not hungry, it is so important. Not only does it start your day off with energy, but it also helps balance your energy and metabolism for the entire day! Skipping breakfast can set you up for food cravings and unhealthy choices later in the day.

2. *Cut down or, even better, eliminate all white processed sugar and flour.* Yes, this includes cakes, cookies, pies, bagels, breads, pastas, etc. Bear in mind that if you eat a lot of processed sugar and carbohydrates, cut back slowly. Your body will go through an easier detox than if you quit cold turkey, and it will be easier for you to stay away from them in the long term.

3. *Watch portion sizes.* Typically, women need only 4–6 ounces of protein with each meal, and men need 6–8 ounces. A serving is equal to the size of the palm of your hand and the thickness of a deck of cards. Americans typically eat way too much protein, especially when dining out. Pay close attention to how much protein you are eating and consider cutting down. Protein sources don't always need to be from animal sources. They can also come from beans, legumes, whole grains, nuts/seeds, and even vegetables, especially the leafy greens. Too much protein can make you sluggish and overweight and can affect your overall health.

4. *Eat vegetables throughout the day.* The low starch vegetables are unlimited! Try to eat a colorful rainbow each day and be sure to include the dark leafy greens each day for optimal nutrition.

5. *Drink pure water (filtered or natural spring water is best).* Our bodies are made up of approximately 2/3 water. Most people drink much less than their daily requirements. If you are not drinking at least 6–8 glasses of water per day, you are probably dehydrated! One sign of dehydration is hunger (your body and mind trick you here), thus leading to weight gain. Other signs include dry skin, fatigue, and joint pain. It is best to drink before and in-between meals. If you don't like the taste of water, add slices of lemon/lime/orange/cucumber, etc., to make it more to your liking. You can also buy flavored water, but make sure it is naturally flavored and that no other ingredients are added.

6. *Exercise.* Any form of exercise is wonderful, not only for your body, but for your mind, as well. Have fun, break it up throughout the day and most of all, don't make it another chore. Some suggested fun exercises include dancing to your favorite music, pulling out your old exercise DVDs, doing gaming exercises on your television, taking brisk walks, hula hooping, or anything that keeps your body moving.

7. *Throw away the scale.* It serves no purpose other than to cause more stress and anxiety. Relating to yourself by a number on a scale is self-defeating. When you do start to exercise, especially with weights, you are building muscle. I am not talking about lifting heavy weights; even with light weights, you can build muscle, which is a good thing. Having lean muscle mass gets fat out of storage. Bear in mind that muscle weighs more than fat. So, weighing yourself is not a true indicator of your weight overall. It is best to take measurements and go by how your clothes fit. If they are getting loose, then you are losing some weight and/or body fat!

8. *Journal.* Either purchase a nice journal or use a pad that you can write in daily. This helps you control what you are eating and also can hold you accountable. Jot down your thoughts and feelings in addition to what you are eating. This will help release bottled-up emotions and help you start to problem solve. Studies show that people who journal lose twice as much weight as those who don't.

I suggest taking the time to let the above tips impact your decision if you really want to lose weight and make your health a priority. Think, what if....

Look beyond a quick fix of just a number on a scale and focus on feeling good, being healthy, having more energy, and feeling fulfilled in all areas of your life. Motivate yourself to get moving and prioritize this motivation as your #1 goal for the year and beyond. It is your life and, ultimately, it is up to you to decide what is really important. Bear in mind that if you don't have your health, you have nothing! Don't fool your-self! Look in the mirror and accept who you are and how you look now. Once you do this, you can slowly make the changes you want to make. Change takes time. Learning something new requires patience with yourself and with your health coach/mentor. Think of it as learning a new language and the start of a new beginning for you towards better health, happiness, and well-being. Weight loss is the end result, and it will be so rewarding to you when you keep it off for more than just a few months!

Choosing foods wisely is helpful to think about. For instance, if you are over-hungry, do you choose a piece of cake, a cookie, chips, or a bagel? What if you had handy and visual to your eye in the fridge an apple, cut-up vegetables, or some protein? Which group do you choose? Notice how you are feeling at the time. Am I stressed, angry, sad, tired, starving, etc., or am I calm, happy, excited, just hungry for a meal? Our moods can dictate which foods we choose at the time. Everything is a choice, and we have to be responsible for our choices. This is why journaling comes in handy; you can see a pattern of the foods you are choosing on a weekly/monthly basis and focus on how you can slowly change those choices to more optimal ones that support you and your health.

We all get food cravings every now and then. Being aware at the time you experience the craving is important. By deconstructing cravings, you can understand what the cravings mean and what our bodies are truly saying and wanting. Getting in touch with our inner-most thoughts and feelings can give us clues as to what we might truly want or need. For example, do we really want that bowl or two of ice cream or piece of cake, or do we really want a hug, a better relationship, a friend to talk to, or an outlet and a calm environment? Is the ice cream or cake replacing what we truly want at the time? Or, it is possible that you might be on a diet that is too restrictive, not allowing for some pleasurable foods? Has enjoyment been taken away from you and your life? Another scenario is that you might be living a stressful, unhappy, and unfulfilling life. When you go out on the weekends, even if alone, try to make it fun. Going to the movies or even renting a DVD is better than sulking and eating out of sadness or frustration. Make friends with yourself again. It is a wonderful, enlightening experience. Relaxing, taking a bath, reading a fun novel, and having some down time just for you are wonderful ways of taking care of yourself. Make time with friends or work colleagues on a weekend in a fun setting where you can let your hair down, laugh, have fun, and be yourself, while at the same time nourishing yourself. When you fight with your spouse, parents, or kids, you might start craving a sweet or salty snack or dessert. Which way do you prefer to be nourished?

Before satisfying a food craving, sit down and take some deep breaths. Perhaps have some water or tea instead. Sometimes cravings are actually due to dehydration. A craving can mean that our bodies are not balanced nutritionally, as well. Instead of reaching for sugary junk foods, try some sweet vegetables, such as a baked sweet potato that has caramelized and tastes almost like candy, or some carrots or sweet fruit. If these options don't work, then go for the craving, but eat it slowly, savoring the flavor, and have just have a small amount. Then the next time you have a craving, remember to try the other suggestions, so make sure you have them on hand. Below I have included a healthy snack list for you to follow when it is impossible to avoid those cravings. The suggestions should be on hand and prepared in advance to keep them as healthy as possible.

There is an old saying from our grandparents' generation: "Food Is Love." Our grandmothers and ancestors cooked well from scratch and, yes, put their "love" into making the food, which is quite important; however, Is Food Really Love? Or has it replaced the love we long for from others, as well as from ourselves? What do we really long for? The more happiness, love, communication, intimacy, connection, peace, freedom, and good health we have in our lives, the less we will focus on food and our cravings. How can you incorporate more of the above into your life? What necessary steps do you need to take in order to have more of these in your life? Take action now rather than wait a few months or years. Time is precious, so don't waste any more time to better yourself and your well-being.

Healthy Snack List

Crunchy
- Lite popcorn, or plain popcorn popped in paper bag in microwave or use coconut oil to pop in a covered pan; best way is hot air popped
- Frozen grapes
- Apple cut up
- Carrots—particularly the super sweet, organic baby carrots
- Crunchy crudités of veggies and hummus or favorite dressing
- Celery and peanut butter (use the non-hydrogenated; hydrogenated fats are plastic fats—not good!) or natural almond butter—1 tablespoon
- Whole grain toast, baby carrots, or rice crackers with hummus
- Dehydrated or baked chick peas with sea salt

Sweet

- Organic carrots or sugar snap peas
- Organic unsweetened yogurt and add your own fruit—all kinds of flavors to enjoy
- Fresh, whole fruit
- Leftover grains (brown rice, quinoa, millet), drizzle raw honey or maple syrup and cinnamon; add almond milk and bananas, heat and enjoy warm oatmeal-like porridge; cook grains in fruit juice, i.e., apple, rice pudding
- Smoothies—mix any of the following (whatever you have in the kitchen): fruit, ice, milk, yogurt, protein powder, carob powder, cocoa powder, fruit juice, etc.
- Frozen yogurt—freeze your own!
- Fruit "ice cream"—peel a banana, freeze, blend in a food processor with nuts, berries, and cocoa powder and serve
- Freshly squeezed veggie juices—make your own and try different combos
- Sweet vegetables—yams, sweet potatoes, squashes (acorn, butternut, kabocha); cut into chunks, sprinkle with cinnamon, add unrefined coconut oil for added flavor and bake
- Dried fruit, mix raw nuts/seeds and dark chocolate chips
- Chia seeds soaked in coconut milk—add berries and some raw honey for a great pudding-like snack

Salty

- Tortilla chips (1 oz.)—try whole grain chips with freshly made salsa or guacamole instead of shelved and processed stuff
- Pickles
- Sauerkraut—it will also knock your sweet craving right out!
- Olives
- Fresh lime/lemon juice as seasonings or in beverage
- Tabbouleh, hummus
- Mixed raw nuts/seeds (make your own trail mix)
- Steamed and lightly salted organic edamame pods

Chewy

- Mochi (pounded sweet rice)—cinnamon raisin is best flavor; add dark chocolate chips to center before cooking for an amazing, yummy snack

*You can find this at some specialty supermarkets and health food stores.

Low-Starch Vegetable List

Artichoke
Artichoke Hearts
Asparagus
Baby Corn
Bamboo Shoots
Beans (green, wax, Italian)
Bean Sprouts
Beet Greens
Brussels Sprouts
Broccoli
Cabbage (green, red, bok choy, Chinese)
Carrots
Cauliflower
Celery
Chayote
Coleslaw (packaged, no dressing)
Cucumber
Daikon
Eggplant
Greens (collard, kale, dandelion, mustard, turnip)
Hearts of Palm

Jicama
Kohlrabi
Leeks
Mushrooms
Okra
Onions
Pea Pods
Peppers
Radishes
Rutabaga
Salad Greens (chicory, endive, escarole, lettuce, romaine, spinach, arugula, radicchio, watercress)
Sprouts
Squash (cushaw, summer, crookneck, spaghetti, zucchini)
Sugar Snap Peas
Swiss Chard
Tomatoes
Turnips
Yard-Long Beans
Zucchini

Chapter 9

Exercise

Why Exercise?

Exercise has many benefits. Here are just a few:

1. Keeps our bodies toned
2. Provides us with endorphins (the feel-good hormone)
3. De-stresses the body by calming it down
4. Gives oxygen to cells, providing more energy to the body
5. Clears our mind
6. Builds self-esteem
7. Prevents muscle loss
8. Strengthens bones
9. Eases back pain
10. Helps prevent diseases

Living a sedentary lifestyle inhibits the above and keeps you from accomplishing your goals. You can easily start exercising at any age, any time, and find the time! Even if you start with just two minutes a day, that is a start to get moving. As a personal fitness trainer, I coach my clients to start slowly and maintain proper form. This is very important. Over the years, I have seen people rush through their workouts, using too much weight and moving too fast when weight training. As a result, they end up hurting themselves unnecessarily. If there is someone to help answer questions at your gym, ask. If no one is available, consider hiring a trainer (a wise investment) for a few sessions to show you how to use the machines correctly and to make sure you are using proper form. If you belong to a gym, I suggest weight training 2–3 times per week for 20–30 minutes. If time permits, you can add an extra day if you want. Start with a short warm-up, and end your workout with some more cardio for 15–20 minutes for beginners and 30–45 minutes for the more advanced. Remember to stretch as well before leaving the gym.

There is no need to overtrain or overexercise. Spending 45 minutes to 1-1/2 hours at the gym is enough, all depending on your level of training.

Even if you don't belong to a gym, you can still exercise. All you need is your mind and body ready for action!

Here are some tips and exercises for you to do at your office/desk and also for your home. I have also included a bonus. For those of you who say you don't have the time to exercise at all, I am sure you can squeeze in 2 minutes in the bathroom, once or twice a day!

Exercise Tips

- Warm up body before exercising by marching in place for 2 minutes (standing or sitting)
- Start slowly and do each exercise with slow, controlled movements to get the most benefit
- Don't hyper-extend your knees or overarch your back
- Engage your abdominal muscles to support your back
- Remember to breathe through each repetition
- Stretch in-between sets and after workouts for injury prevention and flexibility

If you don't have time to go to a gym, I have provided the following exercises and pictures for you to follow. Ideally, it is best to exercise 2–3 times per week, just by doing the exercises given along with some aerobic activity. Don't stress about having to do 30–60 minutes. Start slowly and work your way up to it. Make it fun. Listen to upbeat music while exercising. Let's get going!

Rule of Thumb

For beginners, try to do 1–2 sets of 10–12 repetitions of each exercise.
For the more advanced, do 3 sets of 12–15 repetitions.

Remember to breathe throughout each exercise and repetition. Exhale when you lift, push, or pull through an exercise; inhale during the return of the exercise. This is important to help you obtain each repetition and set without failure and to avoid dizziness or possible fainting.

Here are exercises for you to do at your office/desk, while taking a break!

If you isolate the muscles being worked, you will notice your body weight uses its own resistance.

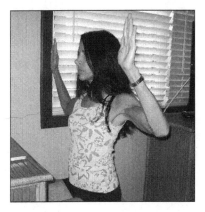 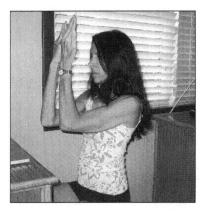

Chest—Chest Press – Strengthens chest and upper body.
- Sit straight with your back against a chair, arms at chest height, elbows bent, shoulder width apart, hands facing each other.
- Slowly move your arms, bringing your forearms together (squeeze your chest muscles, while trying to get your elbows to touch forward); exhale while moving through the exercise. Inhale on the return and repeat.

Back—One-Arm Rows – Strengthens your upper- and mid-back muscles.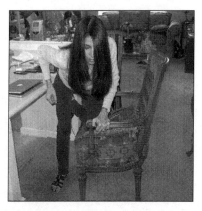
- Rest your left knee on one side of the chair's seat, bend at your waist, lean forward and place your left palm on the side of the seat for support.
- With your right hand, allow your arm to hang down toward the floor in front of the chair with your palm facing the chair.
- Keep a slight bend in your right knee and your right foot flat on the floor.
- Make a fist and pull your arm up in a vertical line into your mid-section, keeping your elbows in close to your torso. (Think pulling weeds out of a garden or starting a lawn mower.)
- Try to squeeze your back muscle just until your hand reaches your chest. Hold this position for a few seconds.
- Exhale when pulling back, inhale on the return and repeat. Then switch sides and repeat.

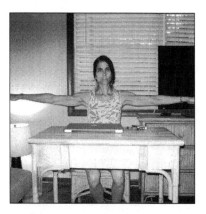 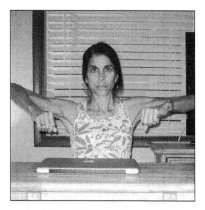

Neck/Shoulders—Arm Circles (above, left)
- Arms should be extended out to each side, parallel to the ground.
- Bring your arms slightly forward, upward, and then backward, making 12 inch circles with your arms.
- Repeat the circle movement and then reverse the motion by going backward, upward, and then forward.

Shoulders—Lateral Raise (above, right)
- Sit in an upright position. Elbows bent at your sides, palms facing towards you.
- Slowly raise your arms, keeping elbows bent, and squeeze the back of your scapula (shoulders). Hold this position for a few seconds. Exhale while lifting; inhale on the return and repeat.

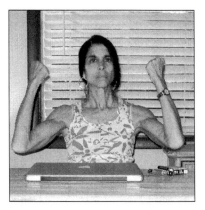

Biceps—Bicep Curl (upper-arm muscles)
- Sit in an upright position, with arms at your sides.
- Make a fist with each hand. Flex your elbows and pull your forearms towards your upper arm (biceps).
- Squeeze your bicep muscles, and hold for a few seconds. Exhale when lifting; inhale on the return and repeat.

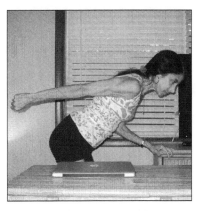 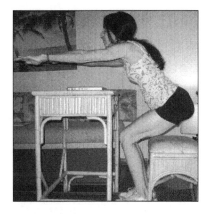

Triceps—Tricep Kickbacks (back of arm muscles) (above, left)
- Rest your left knee on one side of the chair's seat, bend at your waist, lean forward and place your left palm on the side of the seat for support.
- Make a fist with your right hand, palm facing in towards your body and elbow bent.
- Slowly extend your arm back behind you by straightening elbow. Squeeze your tricep muscle (back of your arm), but not fully in locked position, holding for a few seconds, while exhaling.
- Slowly lower back down to starting position. Repeat. After completing one side, switch arms and repeat again. Be sure to keep your wrist straight while doing this exercise.

Thighs & Buttocks—Squats (above, right)
- Place a chair just behind you and stand in front of it with feet about shoulder-width apart.
- Contract your abs and keep them tight as you bend the knees and slowly squat towards the chair.
- Keep the knees behind your toes as you sit down on the chair for a few seconds.
- Contract your glutes and hamstrings to lift up out of the chair and begin extending the legs. Fully extend the legs until you're back to standing position.
- Repeat. To progress, squat down until you're just over the chair, but not sitting all the way down.

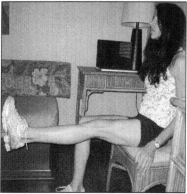

Leg Extension—(upper thigh muscles)
- Sit in an upright position. Hold onto chair for support, legs bent. Straighten left leg, foot flexed.
- Slowly raise leg up as far as it will go, with knee slightly bent (not locked), and squeeze upper thigh muscle. Hold for a few seconds. Then slowly lower leg with control. Repeat.
- After completing one side, switch legs and repeat again.

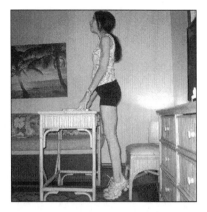 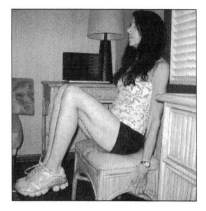

Standing Calf Raises (above, left)
- Stand straight and hold onto desk or wall for stability.
- Slowly come up on your toes as high as possible and hold for a few seconds.
- Slowly lower feet down. Repeat. To progress, do one foot at a time.

Abdominal Crunches (above, right)
- With legs bent, holding onto sides of chair, slowly raise one leg at a time, while squeezing abdominals in and exhaling. Repeat.
- To progress, draw in both legs, tighten abdominals even more to support back, and exhale.

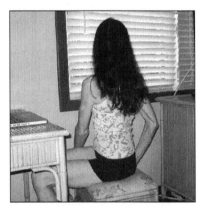 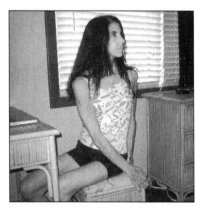

Spinal Rotations—For oblique muscles (inner and outer abs)
- Helps loosen up your lower back and spine. Sit upright in chair.
- Slowly twist your torso to the right and hold for a few seconds. Exhale and then twist to the left.
- Continue twisting your torso slowly, and exhaling.

Stretches at Office/Desk

Hold each stretch for 20–30 seconds

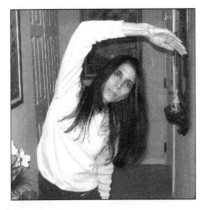 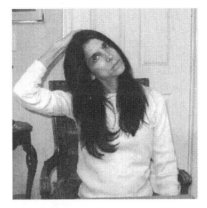

Side Bends (above, left)
While standing, raise right arm straight up and slowly bend to left side of body until you feel a stretch. Switch sides and repeat.

Neck Stretch (above right)
With left arm down at your side, drop head to the right, stretching your neck. Place your right hand on your head and gently press your head into your hand and hold a few seconds. Repeat. Switch sides and repeat.

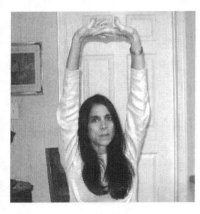

Overhead Stretch (left)
Stand or sit up straight with feet together. With back straight, reach arms straight up and overhead, without locking elbows. You can interlock your fingers and reverse them for a deeper stretch.

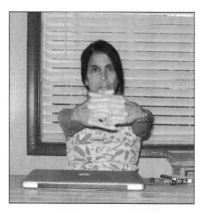 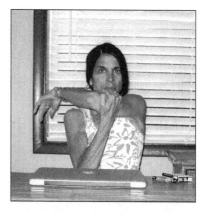

***Chest / Bicep / Shoulder Stretches*)** (above, left)
Stand or sit up straight. Arms out in front of you, clasp hands together and hold. You can interlock your fingers and reverse them for a deeper stretch.

(above, right) Take your left arm straight across your chest and curl the right hand around your elbow, gently pulling on your left arm to deepen the stretch. Switch sides and repeat.

Stand or sit up straight (right). Clasp your hands together behind your back, arms straight. Lift your hands towards the ceiling, going only as high as you are comfortable.

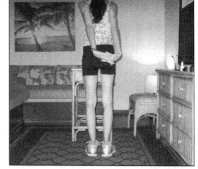

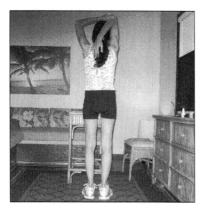

Tricep Stretch (left)
Bend your right elbow behind your head and use your left hand to gently pull your right elbow in further until you feel a stretch in the back of your arm. Switch sides and repeat.

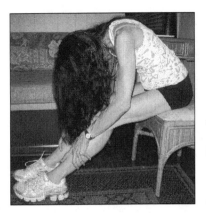

Back Stretch
Hold abs in as you bend forward from the hips, bringing your hands down as close to the floor as possible without being uncomfortable. Relax your head down and reach away from your feet to feel a deep stretch. Inhale and exhale and relax!

Here are exercises you can do at home with some simple equipment using the major muscle groups:

Rule of Thumb

For beginners, start with light weights and try to do 1–2 sets of 10–12 repetitions of each exercise.

For the more advanced, use heavier weights (according to your body and ability) and do 3 sets of 12–15 repetitions. If 15 repetitions are too easy, then slowly increase the weight.

Exercises at Home

A stability ball; 2–4 lb. weights; 5, 7, and 10 lb. dumbbells (higher for those more experienced)

Here are some tips to follow before exercising at home:

- Warm up body before lifting weights by doing 5–8 minutes of cardio (jumping jacks, marching in place, walking, treadmill, or bike is a plus)
- Start slowly and at an easy level
- Don't lift too much weight at once
- Don't hyper-extend your knees or overarch your back
- Engage your abdominal muscles to support your back when lifting
- Remember to breathe through each repetition
- Find an exercise partner who can also help assist when needed
- Consider hiring a personal trainer to show you correct form when lifting weights and just starting out
- Stretch in-between sets and after workout for injury prevention and flexibility

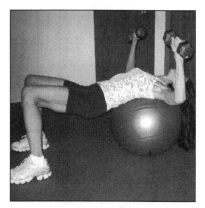 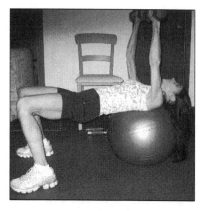

Chest Press on Stability Ball

This exercise utilizes primarily your chest muscles. Assists with shoulders, biceps, and triceps
- With a pair of dumbbells, lie on a stability ball (positioning it underneath your mid to upper back). Keep your feet flat on the floor with your ankles directly under your knees.
- With your hips lifted, engage your core. Holding the dumbbells by your chest, palms facing forward, exhale as you press the weights toward the ceiling. Hold this position for a second or two.
- Slowly lower the weights back to the starting position and repeat—use your abs to keep your body still. Repeat.

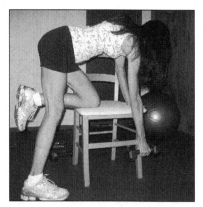 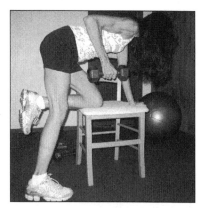

Dumbbell Rows

This exercise utilizes primarily your upper and middle back muscles. Assists with shoulders, biceps and triceps.
- Rest your left knee on one side of the chair's seat. Bend at your waist, lean forward, and place your left palm on the side of the seat for support.
- Grasp your dumbbell with your right hand and allow your arm to hang down toward the floor in front of the chair with your palm facing the chair.
- Keep a slight bend in your right knee and your right foot flat on the floor.
- Bend your right elbow, raise the weight and try squeezing your back muscle just until it reaches your chest. Hold this position for a few seconds. Slowly lower weight towards the floor.
- Repeat. Then switch arms and repeat. (above right)

74 A Whole New You

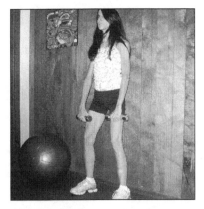 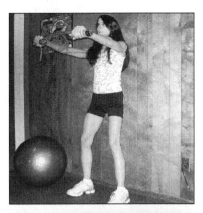

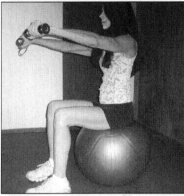

Front Shoulder Raises

- Holding dumbbells in both hands with an overhand grip and palms facing each other, elbows slightly bent, raise both arms directly in front of you until they are parallel with the floor or a little higher.
- Slowly lower weight towards the floor. Repeat. *Note:* you can also do this exercise by raising one arm while the other remains down. It allows you to keep the focus individually on each arm.

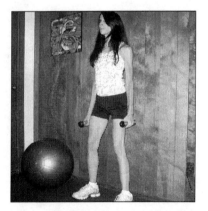 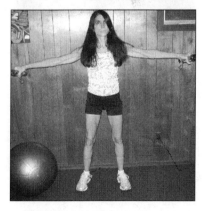

Lateral Shoulder Raises

This exercise is a little more difficult than front shoulder raises.

- Start by using light/medium weights with arms at sides.
- Keeping a slight bend in the elbow, lift the arms out to the sides, stopping at shoulder level. Exhale while lifting weights.
- Make sure you lead with your elbows and not your hands or wrists. Slowly lower weight towards the back of the room. Repeat.

Note: you can do this exercise seated as well. (see photo for seated front shoulder raises).

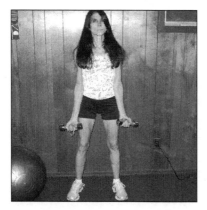 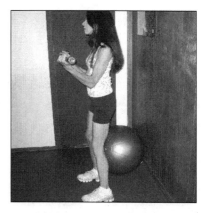

Dumbbell Bicep Curls

- Holding dumbbells in both hands with an underhand grip and palms facing up, elbows slightly bent and at your sides, slowly curl both arms up, squeezing your bicep muscles (front of your arm).
- Hold for a few seconds while exhaling. Slowly lower weight back down, keeping elbows at your sides. Repeat.

Note: you can also do this exercise by raising one arm while the other remains down. It allows you to keep the focus individually on each arm

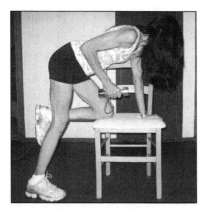 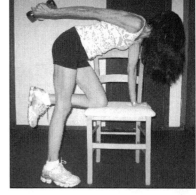

Dumbbell Tricep Kickback

- Rest your left knee on one side of the chair's seat, bend at your waist, lean forward and place your left palm on the side of the seat for support.
- Grasp your dumbbell with your right hand, palm facing in towards your body and elbow bent. Slowly extend the weight back behind you by straightening elbow, squeezing your tricep muscle (back of your arm), but not fully in locked position.
- Hold for a few seconds while exhaling. Slowly lower weight back down to starting position. Repeat.
- After completing one side, switch arms and repeat again. Be sure to keep your wrist straight while doing the exercise.

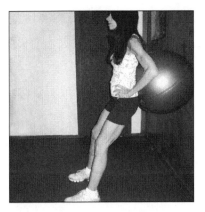 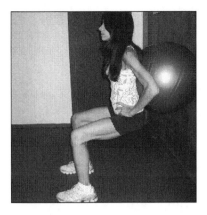

Wall Squats with Stability Ball

This exercise uses primarily your glutes (butt), quadriceps (upper thigh), and hamstring muscles (back of thigh).

- Place ball against a wall and stand with your back against the ball.
- Position the ball into the small of your back. Feet should be shoulder and hip width apart.
- Slowly lower your body as if you are going to sit down in a chair.
- Squeeze your glutes and hold for a few seconds. Be careful not to let the ball roll away from your lower back, and keep feet planted on the floor, utilizing weight on your heels rather than toes.
- Stabilize your core muscles by not leaning too far forward or backward.
- In order to prevent knee injury, it is important that you not let your knees move over your toes. Also, if you have knee pain, don't squat too far down.
- Exhale, slowly pushing your body back up to starting position. Repeat.

Lunges

This is a great exercise for your entire lower body, especially your glutes, hips, and thighs. It is more advanced, so go slowly.

- Stand in a split stance with the left leg forward and the right leg back.
- Your feet should be about 2 to 3 feet apart, depending on your leg length.
- The split stance will require balance, so hold onto a wall or chair if you feel wobbly.
- Before you lunge, make sure that your torso is straight and that you're up on the back toe.
- Bend your knees and lower your body down until your back knee is a few inches from the floor.
- At the bottom of the movement, your front thigh should be parallel to the floor and your back knee should point toward the floor.
- Keep the weight evenly distributed between both legs and push back up, keeping the weight on the heel of your front foot. Repeat. Switch sides and repeat again.

Note: if you have knee issues or feel pain, skip this exercise.

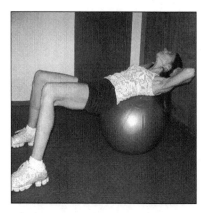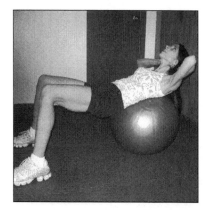

Abdominals on Stability Ball
- Place stability ball about 2 feet in front of wall.
- Lie face up on ball with lower back on its center, knees bent, feet flat on floor, calves parallel to floor.
- Put hands behind head, elbows out to sides. Crunch up; lower. Repeat.

Laura's 2-Minute Exercises in the Bathroom

Yes, you can find the time to exercise, even while you are in the bathroom brushing your teeth! All it takes is 2 minutes, once or twice a day, and over time you will notice your buttocks and thighs getting stronger and leaner! So no more excuses for not exercising!

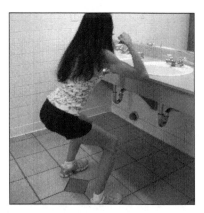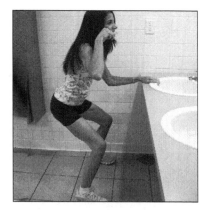

Squats
- Hold onto the side of the sink/vanity with one hand, while brushing teeth with your other hand, feet shoulder and hip-width apart.
- Slowly lower your body as if you are going to sit down in a chair. Squeeze your glutes and hold for a few seconds. Keep feet planted on the floor, utilizing weight on your heels rather than toes. Stabilize your core muscles by not leaning too far forward or back.

In order to prevent knee injury, it is important that you do not let your knees move over your toes. Also, if you have knee pain, don't squat too far down. Exhale, slowly pushing your body back up to starting position.

Note: If balance is an issue, then do this exercise before or after brushing your teeth, but before you leave the bathroom.

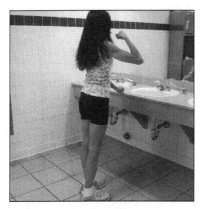 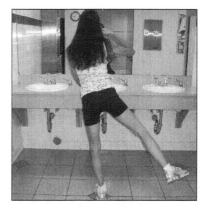

Side Leg Raises
- Hold onto the side of the sink/vanity with one hand, while brushing teeth with your other hand, feet together, standing straight, holding your core in (stomach muscles, not your breath).
- Slowly raise one leg straight out to side, with foot flexed. (Keep opposite leg/knee slightly bent.) It is not necessary to raise your leg high. Avoid bending at the waist to compensate for weak muscles. This exercise is wonderful for strengthening your hips.
- Repeat on opposite leg.

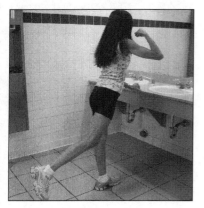

Rear Leg Raises
- Hold onto the side of the sink/vanity with one hand, while brushing teeth with your other hand, feet together, standing straight, holding your core in (stomach muscles, not your breath).
- Slowly raise one leg straight back behind you, with foot flexed. Squeeze glutes and hold for a few seconds. (Keep opposite leg/knee slightly bent.) It is not necessary to raise your leg high.
- Avoid bending at the waist to compensate for weak muscles. This exercise is wonderful for strengthening your hips. Repeat on opposite leg.

Stretching

Stretching is just as important, if not more so, than exercising. As we age, so do our bodies, especially if we skip this step. Our muscles tend to tighten and shorten after we exercise. Focus on lengthening the spine to keep our bodies flexible. If we don't, chronic pain and curvature of the neck, spine, and other parts of the body begin to occur. If you sit at a desk most of the day (especially working at a computer), your upper body, shoulders, and neck tend to lean forward, thus tightening your muscles in these areas. Here are some benefits of stretching:

- Increases blood flow and circulation
- Can improve muscle and joint pain
- Sends oxygen to the brain, calming the mind and body
- Lengthens the spine and other parts of the body

Don't stretch when your body is not warmed up. It's best to stretch after doing some cardiovascular activity or, even better, after you exercise. According to the American College of Sports Medicine (ACSM) guidelines, stretch at least 2–3 times per week and stretch each muscle group using slow, gentle movements. Breathe while you stretch, exhaling as you move into the stretch. Hold the position no more than 20–30 seconds. Three to five repetitions is recommended.

Stretches at Home

Hold each stretch for 20–30 seconds

Chest/Shoulder Stretch
- Sit or stand and clasp your hands together behind your back, arms straight. Lift hands towards the ceiling, going only as high as is comfortable.

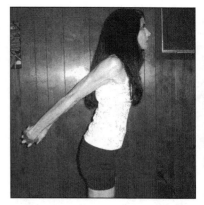

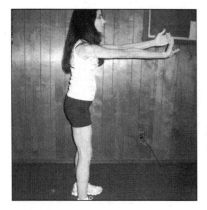

Bicep/Forearm Stretch
- Sit or stand with one arm straight out in front of you, palm up and flexed. Grab onto fingers with left hand and gently pull the fingers back. Repeat with other arm.

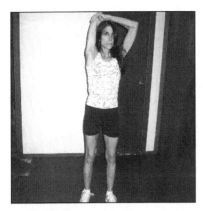

Tricep Stretch

- Bend your right elbow behind your head and use your left hand to gently pull your left elbow until you feel a stretch in the back of your arm (tricep). Repeat with other arm.

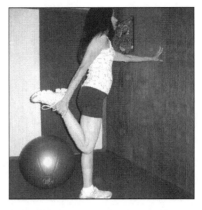

Quadricep Stretch (front of thighs) (right)

- Stand on one foot, holding onto a wall or chair for balance.
- With your free hand, hold onto the back of your ankle. Pull your heel towards your buttocks until you feel a strong stretch in the front of your thigh.

Note: If you can't reach your ankle, place a band or belt around your foot and pull until you feel a strong stretch. Make sure your knee is in line with your hip during stretch.

Another way to do this stretch is by lying on your side on the floor and pulling the opposite leg as stated above.

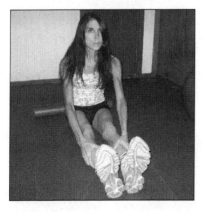

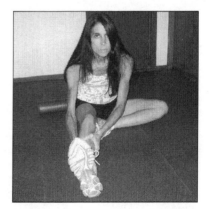

Hamstring Stretch / Forward Bend (back of thigh)

- Sit on the ground with legs straight in front of you. Gently lean forward from the hips (try to keep the back fairly straight) until a stretch is felt on the back of the thighs.
- You can use one leg at a time or both together if more flexible. You can also do this exercise while sitting on a chair, close to the edge or standing with opposite knee bent (do standing only if you have good balance). (continued on page 82)

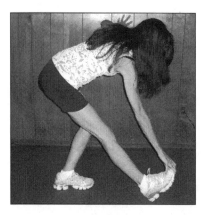

• Straighten right leg, flex foot, and lift heel while leaning forward from your hips. Repeat with other leg.

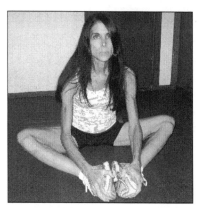

Inner Thigh Stretch (right)
Sit on floor with feet pressed together. Lean forward until you feel a stretch in your inner thighs.

Chapter 10

Stress Reduction

Stress and My Story

Stress reduction is probably the most important aspect of taking care of your health, and many of us make excuses as to why we're not truly focusing on calming our body down and reducing stress (myself included for more than half of my life).

Little did I know that any time my body seemed tense or anxious, I was putting my body in fight or flight mode. I put my adrenal glands into overdrive mostly from stress. My focus was mainly on taking care of my children as a single mother. I didn't realize how much stress can affect your physical body. Mental health feeds physical health and vice versa. My body was worn out. My savior became going to the gym 3–5 times per week. However, I realized later on that too much exercise is not good either. So, when my son was three months old, I decided to go to a yoga class offered at my gym. It was very difficult for the first six months or so. My mind wandered constantly, and I didn't know how to relax my body and mind. I stuck it out and managed to attend one class almost every week. Slowly toward the last 15 minutes of each class, my body seemed to calm down naturally. Using my breath and focusing inward became natural once I got the rhythm and flow of yoga.

I'm glad I pushed myself to keep going and not quit during the first six months, as I have been attending yoga classes once a week for the last 21 years! I can honestly say it is my relaxation time for reflecting, calming my body and mind, stretching, and being at peace. It has become a big part of my life, and being in a class gives me a connection to others. The energy in the room keeps you going, and having a great yoga instructor helps, as well.

Why Is It So Important to Keep the Body Calm?

There are several reasons:

1. ***To keep stress levels down.*** When we're stressed, our body goes into fight or flight mode. We might feel stressed or anxious due to our jobs, school, home life, or even social situations. It seems people are more "stressed out" today than ever. They might experience a faster heart rate, muscle tension, excessive sweating, dryness of mouth, etc. Some people may experience panic attacks, where it might feel like they are having a heart attack or something to that

degree. When we get stressed, over time, our adrenal glands work to release adrenal, our liver releases extra glucose for energy, we might feel sick or tired, and our immune system weakens, as well as many other symptoms.

2. **To control our cortisol levels.** Cortisol is made by the adrenal glands. It helps the body use glucose and use fat for energy (rather than for storage). It also helps manage stress. When cortisol goes up, our bodies tend to store fat rather than burn it and use it for energy, contributing to weight gain or stabilization of weight. Our metabolism essentially shuts down. There is also an increased risk of depression and a quicker aging process.

3. **To reduce diseases.** These include high blood pressure, high cholesterol, diabetes, depression, anxiety, heart disease, weight gain, and obesity, among many others.

4. **To increase sleep and sleep patterns.** Sleep is something most of us don't take as seriously as we should. Lack of sleep increases our stress greatly. When we get five or less hours of sleep a night, our bodies don't get the REM sleep we need. Some people think having a glass or two of wine or beer close to bedtime will help with sleep; however, after a few hours, your body awakens and is more stressed than it was originally. Over time, the alcohol and the sugar in it take a toll on your body. Then, in the morning, you function by having caffeine and/or sugar to keep you awake. Our bodies need 7–8 hours of sleep per night to function optimally. The latest you should go to bed is 10–11pm at least five days a week. Otherwise, your sleep cycle gets interrupted and your organs cannot work to detoxify properly. In addition, your cortisol levels might rise, and you might experience a second or even third wind, all depending on the time you go to sleep. If you tend to go to sleep in the wee hours of the morning, have you noticed that it is more difficult to fall asleep?

What Does Stress Do to Our Bodies?

Stress is the body's natural way of protecting itself. However, when we are in a constant state of stress (chronic), our bodies can exhibit many physical, as well as emotional, symptoms. Our muscles can be in a constant state of tension, which can lead to headaches and muscle tension in the upper body, such as in the neck, head, and shoulders. It can also lead to back pain, causing many physical symptoms in the back and spine.

Stress can affect the cardiovascular system in our bodies. It can affect our heart rate by increasing the amount of blood to parts of the body and elevating blood pressure. This is also known as the fight or flight response. Long-term ongoing stress can increase the risk of hypertension, heart attack, or even stroke.

When our bodies are stressed, a process is started to produce epinephrine and cortisol (also known as the stress hormones). When these hormones are released, the liver produces more glucose (a blood sugar that gives more energy for a fight or flight) in an emergency to the body. For some people, the blood sugar does not get reabsorbed in the body if not used, and can cause Type 2 diabetes.

Stress can make us eat more or less than we normally do. It can affect our digestion and absorption of nutrients. Heartburn, reflux, and even stomach ulcers can occur. We might also choose to drink alcohol, smoke, or take drugs, leading to other complications in our body.

Stress can affect our sleep patterns and behaviors, as well. When we are stressed, we tend to either sleep too much or too little. Having a balance and trying to get at least 7–8 hours of sleep per night is essential.

Stress can affect our minds. It can contribute to lack of concentration, constant worrying, anxiousness, and poor judgement. We might feel irritable, moody, overwhelmed, agitated and unable to relax, lonely, and even depressed.

It is important to make the time to learn how to de-stress the mind and body.

Recommended Stress-Reduction Techniques:

Yoga

Yoga was first discovered and written in India centuries ago. The Yogic System was first codified, or put into writing, by Patanjali in "The Yoga Sutras." The Sutras were short verses known as the Royal Path or the Eight Limbs of Yoga. They are believed to have been compiled around 400 BC. The third limb is known as the asanas, where yogis use their yoga practice for postures to keep the body flexible and disease-free. The great Paramhansa Yogananda was sent to the U.S. from India in 1920 to share the teachings of yoga in the West. Yoga is now well-known throughout the U.S. and the world as a wonderful form of exercise and relaxation.

Yoga is a state of individual consciousness and universal state of being. Its original purpose was to prepare for meditation. In modern times, yoga had been used to find inner peace and fulfillment, and to achieve flexibility, calmness, and overall better health.

Benefits
- Flexibility
- Builds Muscle & Core Strength
- Lengthens Spine
- Better Posture
- Increases Relaxation for the Body and Mind
- Decreases Blood Pressure
- Inner Peace
- Better Focus and many other benefits!

Mindfulness Based Stress Reduction

What is it? *Mindfulness is the practice of purposely focusing your attention on the present moment—and accepting it without judgment.*

Mindfulness Based Stress Reduction, also known as MBSR, is a balance of meditation, body awareness, and yoga.

The MBSR program originally was conceived to help medical patients manage stress associated with medically challenging conditions, initially focusing on chronic pain. One of the founders, Jon Kabat-Zinn, discovered that focusing on the present moment and practicing mindfulness rather than focusing on the physical or emotional pain a patient was feeling helped them. He noted that a significant amount of the pain was reduced. It sounds simpler to do than it might be. It may open some experiences of pain and other experiences we might tend to avoid. Mindfulness practice proposes to relieve suffering and advocates acceptance as a core attitude. Not practicing the technique, however, can keep us in the original state we were in. Over time, it will get easier as long as it is practiced.

Mindfulness helps you train your mind to concentrate in the moment, rather than do many things or have many thoughts at once. It helps you focus on the present moment, and not the day-to-day stresses or worries about the past or future. I believe this type of practice is essential for all to do. It only needs to take a few minutes a day. If your mind wanders and thoughts come up, notice them, let them pass—like a cloud in the sky—and gently redirect yourself back to the present moment. I practice mindfulness a few minutes each day. It is a good idea to schedule a few minutes into your day, as well. I never thought I would be able to do this, as my brain is always thinking, doing, multitasking, etc. I think that taking up yoga has helped with this notion. Yoga, as previously discussed, is the stepping stone to meditation. Learning to quiet the mind and body is not easy for most of us, but starting slowly with yoga, listening to soft music, or being in nature is quite helpful. It helps you focus inward on your true self.

Benefits
- Stress Reduction
- Improves Sleep
- Lowers Blood Pressure
- Helps Obsessive Compulsive Disorder
- Helps Lower Anxiety & Depression
- Helps with Eating Disorders

For a wonderful resource to a free on-line 8-week program, go to: www.palousemindfulness.com.

Meditation

Quietly sitting in a comfortable position and letting your body, mind, emotions, and energy focus on your inner-self will bring you into a meditative state naturally. The key is to be in control of your mind rather than your mind being in control of you and your thoughts. Many people, including myself, find it rather difficult to sit for long periods of time and focus on breathing. Using a mantra, word, or number repeated over and over again helps you focus inwardly. Some examples are "om" or "I am" or "peace" or "love." For beginners, count while breathing through your nostrils by inhaling to the count of 1, then exhaling to the count of 1, inhaling to the count of 2, then exhaling to the count of 2, and so on until you finish to the count of 10. Repeat 2 or 3 rounds of counting to 10 while using your breath. The more you practice, the better able you will be to control your mind and the chatter that goes on.

Benefits
- Quiets the Mind and Body
- De-stresses the Body
- Increases Happiness
- Helps Immune System
- Gain Insight and Clarity
- Deeper Connection to Oneself
- Increases Overall Health and Well-Being

Visualization

Close your eyes and visualize a time in your life that was memorable and happy. Maybe it was a vacation, outing, or just relaxing with a loved one. Focus your mind and body as if you were there at that moment. Focus and breathe and relax into it. Enjoy the peace and calm you are feeling. Try to stay focused for at least 10 minutes in this relaxed state of mind. Come out of the visualization slowly when ready, and take note in your mind's eye throughout the day of how the visualization made you feel. It has been noted that using this technique before surgery can help one cope with the stress of surgery and/or anesthesia.

Positive Affirmations

They are statements or quotes that increase positive self-talk. Affirmations can be spoken or written. If spoken, it is best to repeat the affirmations at least 25 times in the morning (upon waking) and in the evening (before bedtime). They are the optimal times to practice. Saying the affirmation in front of the mirror is very effective. Saying them out loud or to yourself during the course of the day is an added plus. You can also write down the affirmations, if that is easier for you, at a minimum of 20 times per day—10 times upon waking in the morning and 10 times before bedtime. You can also write down each affirmation on an index card to carry with you and review 20 times per day. The more you practice, the more beneficial it will be. Pick the best way for you and be consistent!

I came across a wonderful website that has 100 positive affirmations, grouped according to how you are feeling at the time. Affirmations are best used in the present tense. Check out this website for some wonderful affirmations: http://www.self-help-and-self-development.com/affirmations.html

Benefits
- Positive Mindset
- Greater Confidence
- Creates Happiness Feelings
- Creates Abundance in Your Life

Here are a few positive affirmations to remember or post on your refrigerator or mirror:

- I love myself unconditionally and accept myself as I am.
- I surround myself with people who treat me well.
- I take the time to show my friends/family that I care about them.
- I see the perfection in all my flaws.
- I feel good only when I eat wholesome, natural food. Junk food makes me feel unwell.
- Every passing day, my body becomes more energetic and healthier.
- I enjoy the challenge of a meaningful, worthwhile goal.
- I can do it.

References

Chapter 2

Griffin, R. Morgan, and Brunilda Nazario. *"Healthy Whole Foods: Making Nutrient-Rich Choices for Your Diet."* WebMD, 12 May 2009. Web. 23 Feb. 2015.

"Enjoy a Moment of Calm." Calm.com. N.p., Mar. 2012. Web. 30 Mar. 2015.

Chapter 3

"No More Emotional Baggage." Ether: FAQ About Emotional Baggage. PWM Program, 4 Sept. 2010. Web. 23 Feb. 2015.

Chapter 5

Robbins, John, and Ocean Robbins. *"Join the FREE Healthy Kitchen Power Hour with John and Ocean Robbins."* Food Revolution Network. N.p., 2014. Web. 27 Feb. 2015.

Chapter 6

Lehman, Shereen, MS. *"Quinoa—Andean Superfood."* About Health. About.com, 07 Jan. 2015. Web. 19 Mar. 2015.

"EWG's Shopper's Guide to Pesticides in Produce™." *EWG's 2015 Shopper's Guide to Pesticides in Produce™.* Environmental Working Group, 2015. Web. 02 Apr. 2015.

Chapter 8

Rosenthal, Joshua. *Deconstructing Cravings.* New York: Institute For Integrative Nutrition, Nov. 2004. PDF.

"Non-starchy Vegetables." American Diabetes Association. American Diabetes Association, 14 May 2014. Web. 31 Mar. 2015.

Chapter 9

Bibb, Emily. *"Back to Basics: Stability Ball Chest Press."* RSS. POPSUGAR, 09 Oct. 2013. Web. 03 Apr. 2015.

Howard, Michelle M. *"Whole Body Dumbbell Workout Using a Chair."* Healthy Living. Demand Media, n.d. Web. 03 Apr. 2015.

Miller, P.T., Ph.D, FACSM, Lynn. *"Improving Your Flexibility and Balance."* ACSM I Articles. ACSM. org, 02 Feb. 2012. Web. 28 Feb. 2015.

Waehner, Paige. *"Strength Training and Specialty Workouts."* About Health. About.com, 2015. Web. 02 Apr. 2015.

Chapter 10

Tovian, PhD, Steven, Beverly Thom, PhD., Helen Coons, PhD., Susan Labott, PhD, Matt Burg, PhD, Richard Surwit, PhD, and Daniel Bruns, PsyD. *"Stress Effects on the Body."* Http://www.apa.org. American Psychological Association, Jan. 2014. Web. 25 Feb. 2015.

Yogananda, Paramhansa. Autobiography of a Yogi. N.d. TS. Ananda Sangha Worldwide. Crystal Clarity Publishers, 2009. Web. 28 Feb. 2015.

Carrico, Mara. *"Learn the Eight Limbs of Yoga | Yoga Philosophy | Yoga for Beginners."* Yoga Journal. Cruz Bay Publishing, Inc., 28 Aug. 2007. Web. 27 Feb. 2015.

Siegel, Psy.D., Ronald D., and Steven M. Allison, Psy.D.: *Practices for Improving Emotional and Physical Well-Being.* Rep. Harvard Health Publications, 2013. Web. 28 Feb. 2015.

"Benefits of Mindfulness." Helpguide.org. Helpguide.org, 2013. Web. 11 Feb. 2015. ©Helpguide.org. All rights reserved. Helpguide.org is a non-profit guide to better mental and emotional health.

Potter, Dave. *"Palouse Mindfulness."* Palouse Mindfulness. Dave Potter, n.d. Web. 31 Mar. 2015.

Vishwasrao, Prasanna. *"Affirmations."* Http://www.self-help-and-self-development.com/. Prasanna Vishwasrao, 2005. Web. 28 Feb. 2015.